THE PEGAN DIET

EMPHASIZE NUTRIENT-RICH FRUITS, VEGETABLES, HEALTHY FATS FROM PLANTS AND NATURALLY GROW ANIMALS FOR PREVENT DISEASE, REDUCE INFLAMMATION AND PROMOTE HEART HEALTH

ANIYHA KEYS

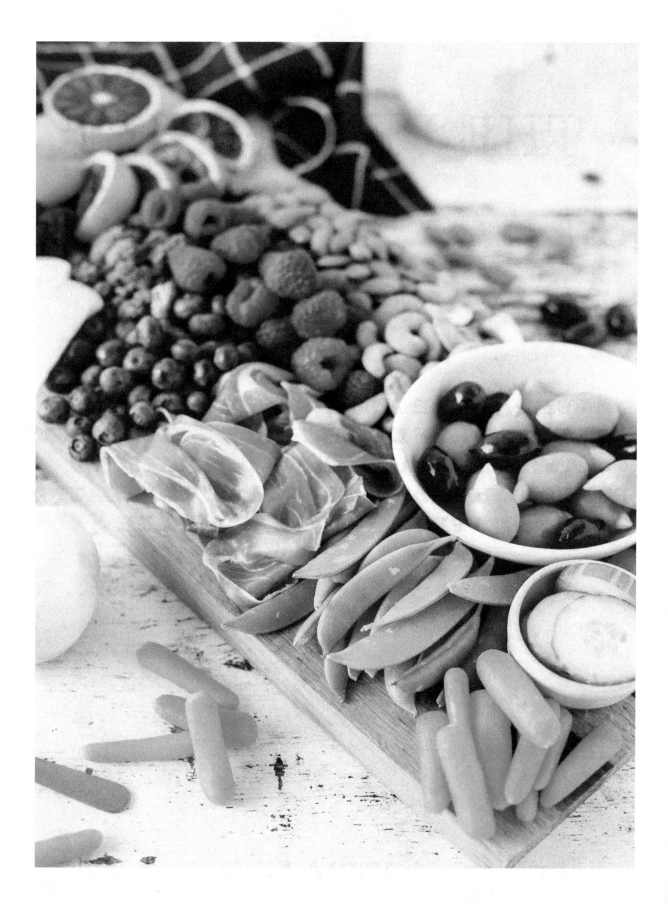

Introduction

The Pegan Diet is a worldwide trending diet that owes its spread to its mysterious origin. Its true roots combine certain aspects of two diets - Paleo and Vegan, which don't add up well on paper. The term Pegan was coined by Dr. Mark Hyman, the director of the Cleveland Clinic Centre for Functional Medicine, who claims that the Pegan way of eating is not only the most sensible diet designed for the human race, but it is also the healthiest.

Pegan Diet includes about 50% of plant foods (fruits, vegetables and whole grains) that are low in calories but high in nutrition. The other 50% is rich in proteins from plants, healthy fats from nuts, seeds, fish and seafood and low-fat dairy products. In a word, Pegan Diet contains more nutrients rather than calories. Therefore, it will never make you obese or overweight because it has a low-calorie density (grams of calories per 100 grams).

Adopting Pegan Diet can help you to achieve an ideal weight without going through any kind of strict and hard dieting. This is because 1) Pegan Diet contains more fiber than any other diet. Fiber makes you feel full in addition fulfilled so that you don't need to take a large portion of food. 2) Pegan Diet contains various plant foods from which you can select the ones that will be favorable to you. For example, if you like apples and oranges but dislike broccoli, you can easily make a choice. 3) Pegan Diet is designed to help you burn more calories than any other diet. This is because it contains both kinds of nutrients: fats and carbohydrates. When your body burns the nutrients for energy, it will produce heat. The larger the number of nutrients, the more heat will be produced and in turn more calories will be burned.

Pegan Diet can provide your body with adequate nutrition for both brain and gut health.

The brains are made with 60% fats. Pegan Diet can improve your brain health in two ways: (1) it contains a sufficient amount of omega 3 fatty acids, which are essential for the healthy function of the brain; (2) it includes nuts, seeds, legumes and whole grains which are excellent sources of vegetable protein and healthy fats.

Pegan Diet can improve your memory power and brain function generally; enhance gut health to promote healthy digestion and break down of undigested food in the intestines; reduce skin inflammation in acne patients; protect against eczema by stopping the chain of inflammatory reactions in skin cells. How does it improve your gut health? Pegan Diet contains two kinds of fiber: soluble fiber (found in fruits, vegetables, nuts and legumes, especially oats) and insoluble fiber (found in whole grains). Soluble fiber helps reduce the risk of diverticulosis and diverticulitis. Insoluble fiber reduces constipation.

Pegan Diet can reduce the risk of inflammatory bowel disease by reducing intestinal permeability; improve bowel movements and treat diarrhea; help to prevent colon cancer.

Pegan Diet can promote gastric ulcer healing; decrease the incidence of gallstones; cure itchy skin conditions like atopic dermatitis (eczema), urticaria (hives) and psoriasis.

The Vegan Diet

A Vegan diet is built on a certain set of strict rules, with the primary rule prohibiting the consumption of all animal products and giving most importance to plant-based foods. This diet lacks meat and other rich sources of bio-molecules like dairy and eggs. Most vegans are extremely careful about what they consume. Apart from the restrictions mentioned above, they also avoid processed animal products like gelatin, which is often added to foods, even those that seem vegan.

The resulting diet is essentially one low in calories, cholesterol, and saturated fat. This can be very beneficial for anyone who wants faster weight loss. It is also good for those with heart conditions, as it assists in cholesterol and blood pressure regulation. Vegan as a diet is getting increasingly accepted due to its many health benefits.

The Paleo Diet

The Paleo Diet has been around for centuries, having originated in The Paleolithic era. Its followers were the ancient people of the Stone Age. As a predecessor, the Paleo diet uses only food available to our ancestors and eliminates or restricts modern foods. The paleo diet involves a higher level of consumption of meat and vegetables with a very light sprinkling of fruits and nuts. Additions and alternatives like grains, beans, added sugar, dairy and several kinds of oils are to be avoided.

By way of comparison, the founders of the paleo diet, the cave people, consumed foods that were hunted by our hunter ancestors and included grass-fed meat, fish, eggs, nuts, fruit, and organic low-starch vegetables. Although the fat content isn't restricted, foods like grains, legumes, refined sugar, potatoes, most dairy products, and certain oils are prohibited. On the contrary, a vegan diet is heavily based on plant food consumption. Their diet consists of vegetables, fruits, grains, nuts, and seeds while strictly prohibiting any form of animal product.

Most Paleo dieters have small portions of meat included with every meal. This means that approximately 30-50% of a person's daily energy is obtained through the meat. These levels are twice the number when compared to current nutrition guidelines that fluctuate around 15% to 25% of a day's energy obtained through the meat.

Chapter 1.   14 Pillars Of Pegan Diet

The Pegan Diet is similar to the Paleo Diet in that it does not allow refined carbs, processed foods or dairy products. It is also similar to the Ketogenic Diet in that it does not allow gluten or added sugars. The Pegan Diet is different from both of these diets because it allows for higher carbohydrate intake than either.

Here are the 14 pillars of the pegan diet

1. Consume foods that are high in healthy fats. I'm speaking about omega-3 fatty acids also other healthy fats found in nuts, beans, olive oil, and avocados, to name a few. Yes, saturated fat from fish, whole eggs, grass-fed or sustainably raised beef, grass-fed butter or ghee, and coconut butter or organic virgin coconut oil are all acceptable sources of saturated fat.

2. Avoid most, nut, and seed oils, including canola, sunflower, corn, grapeseed, and soybean oil, which now account for around 10% of our calories. Small quantities of expeller or cold-pressed nut and seed oils, such as sesame, macadamia, and walnut, can be used as condiments or flavorings. Avocado oil is suitable for cooking at higher temperatures.

3. Limit or exclude dairy. Dairy isn't good for most people, so I suggest avoiding it, with the exception of kefir, yogurt, ghee, grass-fed butter, and even cheese if it does not bother you. Instead of cow dairy, try goat or sheep dairy. Also, go organic and grass-fed whenever possible.

4. Consider meat and animal products as a side dish, or as I like to refer to them, "condi-meat," rather than the main course. Meat should be a side dish, with vegetables taking center stage. Per meal, servings should be no more than 4 to 6 ounces. I usually prepare three or four vegetable side dishes at a time.

5. Consume low-mercury fish that has been sustainably raised or harvested. Choose low-mercury and low-toxin seafood such as sardines, herring, anchovies, and wild-caught salmon if you're eating fish (all of which have high omega-3 and low mercury levels).

6. Stay away from gluten. Wheat can only be eaten if you are not gluten-intolerant, and even then, only on special occasions.

7. Avoid sugar at all costs. That means avoiding sugar, starch, and refined carbohydrates, all of which cause an increase in insulin output. Consider sugar in all of its types as a once-in-a-while indulgence, something we consume in moderation. People should think of it as a recreational drug, I tell them. It's something you do for fun now and then, but it's not something you eat every day.

8. Eat predominantly plant-based foods. Vegetables can occupy more than half of your plate, as we learned earlier. The better the hue, the darker it is. The greater the range, the better. Stop starchy vegetables as far as possible. In moderation (12 cups per day), winter squashes and sweet potatoes are perfect. There aren't enough potatoes! Even though French fries are America's most common vegetable, they don't count.

9. Taking it easy on the fruits. This is where there might be some misunderstanding. Some Paleo advocates advise consuming only low-sugar fruits including berries, while vegan advocates advise eating all fruit. Many of my patients seem to feel happier when they stick to low-glycemic fruits and treat themselves to the rest. Stick to bananas, kiwis, and watermelon, and avoid oranges, melons, and other similar fruits. Consider dried fruit to be sweets, and use it sparingly.

10. Avoid pesticides, antibiotics, hormones, and genetically modified crops. Additionally, there are no pesticides, oils, preservatives, dyes, artificial sweeteners, or other potentially harmful ingredients. You should not eat an ingredient if you do not have it in your kitchen for cooking. Anyone for polysorbate 60, red dye 40, and sodium stearoyl lactylate (a.k.a. Twinkie ingredients)?

11. Consume gluten-free whole grains in moderation. They also increase blood sugar and have the ability to cause autoimmunity. A grain- and bean-free diet can be crucial for type 2 diabetics, as well as those with autoimmune disease or digestive disorders, in treating and even reversing their illness.

12. Just eat beans once in a while. The best legume is lentils. Big, starchy beans should be avoided. Beans have a high fiber, protein, and mineral content. However, for some people, they cause digestive issues, and the lectins and phytates in them can inhibit mineral absorption. If you have diabetes, a high-bean diet will cause blood sugar spikes.

13. Get your solution checked so you can adapt it to your unique needs. What is effective for one individual might not be effective for another. This is what I mean when I say that everyone can eventually work with a functionally qualified nutritionist to personalize their diet even further with the right tests.

14. Stay away from booze and coffee.

Chapter 2.   Breakfast

Paleo Banana Pancakes

Preparation Time: 5 Minutes

Cooking Time: 5 Minutes

Servings: 2

Ingredients:

- A pinch of salt

- Two bananas, peeled and chopped

- ¼ tsp. baking powder

- Cooking spray

Directions:

1. In a bowl, mix the chopped bananas, a pinch of salt and baking powder and whisk well.
2. Transfer this to your food processor and blend very well.
3. Heat up a pan over medium high heat after you've sprayed it with some cooking oil.
4. Add some of the pancakes batter, spread in the pan, cook for 1 minute, flip and cook for 30 seconds and transfer to a plate.
5. Serve and enjoy!

Nutrition:

Calories: 120

Fat: 2g

Carbs: 2g

Protein: 4g

Fiber: 6.6g

Sugar: 1g

Orange and Dates Granola

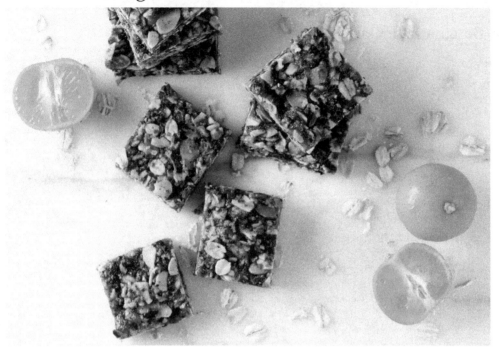

Preparation Time: 5 Minutes

Cooking Time: 25 Minutes

Servings: 6

Ingredients:

- 5 oz. dates, soaked in hot water

- Juice from 1 orange

- Grated rind of ½ orange

- 1 cup desiccated coconut

- ½ cup silvered almonds

- ½ cup pumpkin seeds

- ½ cup linseeds

- ½ cup sesame seeds

- Almond milk for serving

Directions:

1. In a bowl, mix almonds with orange rind, orange juice, linseeds, coconut, pumpkin and sesame seeds and stir well.

2. Drain dates, add them to your food processor and blend well.

3. Add this paste to almonds mix and stir well again.

4. Spread this on a lined baking sheet, introduce in the oven at 350 degrees and bake for 15 minutes, stirring every 4 minutes.

5. Take granola out of the oven, leave aside to cool down a bit and then serve with almond milk.

6. Enjoy!

Nutrition:

Calories: 208

Fat: 9g

Carbs: 3g

Protein: 6g

Fiber: 5g

Sugar: 0g

Green Breakfast Smoothie

Preparation Time: 10 minutes

Cooking time: 0 minutes

Servings: 2

Ingredients:

- 1/2 Banana, sliced
- 2 cups spinach
- 1 cup sliced berries of your choosing, fresh or frozen
- 1 orange, peeled and cut into segments
- 1 cup unsweetened nondairy milk
- 1 cup ice

Directions:

1. In a blender, combine all the ingredients.
2. Starting with the blender on low speed, begin blending the smoothie, gradually increasing blender speed until smooth. Serve immediately.

Nutrition:

Calories: 208;

Fat: 8g;

Protein: 14g;

Carbohydrates: 22g;

Fiber: 7g;

Sugar: 1g;

Sodium: 596mg

Warm Maple and Cinnamon Quinoa

Preparation Time: 5 minutes

Cooking time: 15 minutes

Servings: 4

Ingredients:

- 1 cup unsweetened nondairy milk
- 1 cup water
- 1 cup quinoa, rinsed
- 1 teaspoon cinnamon
- 1/4 cup chopped pecans
- 2 tablespoons pure maple syrup or agave

Directions:

1. Bring the almond milk, water, and quinoa to a boil. Lower the heat to medium-low and cover. Cook gently until the quinoa softens, about 15 minutes.
2. Turn off the heat and allow sitting, covered, for 5 minutes. Stir in the cinnamon, pecans, and syrup. Serve hot.

Nutrition:

Calories: 110;

Fat: 9g;

Protein: 15g;

Carbohydrates: 25g;

Fiber: 7g;

Sugar: 4g;

Sodium: 210mg

Blueberry and Chia Smoothie

Preparation Time: 10 minutes

Cooking time: 0 minutes

Servings: 2

Ingredients:

- 2 tablespoons chia seeds
- 2 cups unsweetened nondairy milk
- 2 cups blueberries, fresh or frozen
- 2 tablespoons pure maple syrup or agave
- 2 tablespoons cocoa powder

Directions:

1. Blend together the soaked chia seeds, almond milk, blueberries, maple syrup, and cocoa powder and blend until smooth. Serve immediately

Nutrition:

Calories: 100;

Fat: 18g;

Protein: 19g;

Carbohydrates: 20g;

Fiber: 9g;

Sugar: 4g;

Sodium: 500mg

Apple and Cinnamon Oatmeal

Preparation Time: 5 minutes

Cooking time: 15 minutes

Servings: 4

Ingredients:

- 1/4 cups apple cider
- 1 apple, peeled, cored, and chopped
- 2/3 cup rolled oats
- 1 teaspoon ground cinnamon
- 1 tablespoon pure maple syrup

Directions:

1. Take the apple cider to a boil over medium-high heat. Stir in the apple, oats, and cinnamon.
2. Bring the cereal to a boil and turn down heat to low. Simmer until the oatmeal thickens, 3 to 4 minutes. Spoon into two bowls and sweeten with maple syrup, if using. Serve hot.

Nutrition:

Calories: 110;

Fat: 9g;

Protein: 15g;

Carbohydrates: 25g;

Fiber: 7g;

Sugar: 4g;

Sodium: 210mg

Spiced Orange Breakfast Couscous

Preparation Time: 5 minutes

Cooking time: 15 minutes

Servings: 4

Ingredients:

- 3 cups orange juice
- 1.1/2 cups couscous
- 1 teaspoon ground cinnamon
- 1/4 teaspoon ground cloves
- 1/2 cup dried fruit
- 1/2 cup chopped almonds

Directions:

1. Take the orange juice to a boil. Add the couscous, cinnamon, and cloves and remove from heat. Shield the pan and allow sitting until the -couscous softens.
2. Fluff the couscous and stir in the dried fruit and nuts. Serve -immediately. Pecans and syrup. Serve hot.

Nutrition:

Calories: 110;

Fat: 9g;

Protein: 15g;

Carbohydrates: 25g;

Fiber: 7g;

Sugar: 4g;

Sodium: 210mg

Broiled Grapefruit with Cinnamon Pitas

Preparation Time: 5 minutes

Cooking time: 15 minutes

Servings: 4

Ingredients:

- 2 whole-wheat pitas cut into wedges

- 2 tablespoons coconut oil, melted

- 1 tablespoon ground cinnamon

- 2 tablespoons brown sugar

- 1 grapefruit, halved

- 2 tablespoons pure maple syrup or agave

Directions:

1. Preheat the oven to 375°F. Line a baking sheet with parchment paper.
2. Spread pita wedges in a single layer on a baking sheet and brush with melted coconut oil.
3. In a small bowl, combine the cinnamon and brown sugar and sprinkle over the pita wedges.
4. Bake in preheated oven until the wedges are crisp, about 8 minutes. Transfer the pita wedges to a plate and set aside.
5. Turn the oven to broil. Drip the maple syrup over the top of the grapefruit, if using. Broil until the syrup bubbles and begins to crystallize, 3 to 5 minutes. Serve immediately.

Nutrition:

Calories: 115;

Fat: 19g;

Protein: 25g;

Carbohydrates: 35g;

Fiber: 17g;

Sugar: 14g;

Sodium: 210mg

Breakfast Parfaits

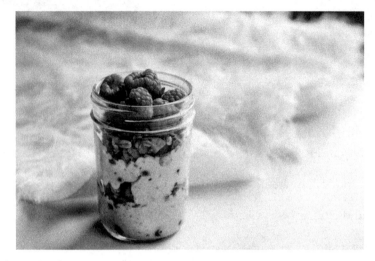

Preparation Time: 5 minutes

Cooking time: 15 minutes

Servings: 4

Ingredients:

- One 14-ounce cans coconut milk, refrigerated overnight

- 1 cup granola

- 1/2 cup walnuts

- 1 cup sliced strawberries or other seasonal berries

Directions:

1. Pour off the canned coconut-milk liquid and retain the solids.
2. In two parfait glasses, layer the coconut-milk solids, granola, walnuts, and -strawberries. Serve immediately.

Nutrition:

Calories: 125;

Fat: 9g;

Protein: 15g;

Carbohydrates: 35g;

Fiber: 17g;

Sugar: 18g;

Orange French toast

Preparation Time: 5 minutes

Cooking time: 15 minutes

Servings: 4

Ingredients:

- 3 very ripe bananas
- 1 cup unsweetened nondairy milk
- Zest and juice of 1 orange
- 1 teaspoon ground cinnamon
- 1/4 teaspoon grated nutmeg
- 4 slices French bread
- 1 tablespoon coconut oil

Directions:

1. Blend the bananas, almond milk, orange juice and zest, cinnamon, and nutmeg and blend until smooth. Dip the bread in the mixture for 5 minutes on each side.
2. While the bread soaks, heat a griddle or sauté pan over medium-high heat. Melt the coconut oil in the pan and swirl to coat. Cook the bread slices until golden brown on both sides, about 5 minutes each. Serve immediately.

Nutrition:

Calories: 113;

Fat: 19g;

Protein: 25g;

Carbohydrates: 85g;

Fiber: 19g;

Sugar: 18g;

Sodium: 320mg

Pumpkin Pancakes

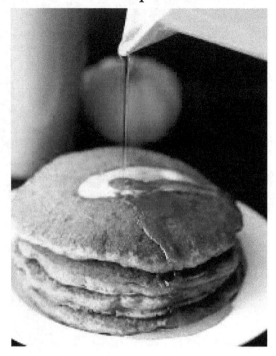

Preparation Time: 5 minutes

Cooking time: 15 minutes

Servings: 4

Ingredients:

- 2 cups unsweetened almond milk
- 1 teaspoon apple cider vinegar
- 2.1/2 cups whole-wheat flour
- 2 tablespoons baking powder
- 1/2 teaspoon baking soda
- 1 teaspoon sea salt
- 1 teaspoon pumpkin pie
- 1/2 cup canned pumpkin purée
- 1 cup water
- 1 tablespoon coconut oil

Directions:

1. Dip together the flour, baking powder, baking soda, salt and pumpkin pie spice.

2. In another large bowl, combine the almond milk mixture, pumpkin purée, and water, whisking to mix well.

3. Add the wet ingredients to the dry ingredients and fold together until the dry -ingredients are just moistened. You will still have a few streaks of flour in the bowl.

4. In a nonstick pan or griddle over medium-high heat, melt the coconut oil and swirl to coat. Pour the batter into the pan 1/4 cup at a time and cook until the pancakes are browned, about 5 minutes per side. Serve immediately.

Nutrition:

Calories: 113;

Fat: 19g;

Protein: 25g;

Carbohydrates: 85g;

Fiber: 19g;

Sugar: 18g;

Sodium: 320mg

Sweet Potato and Kale Hash

Preparation Time: 10 minutes

Cooking time: 15 minutes

Servings: 2

Ingredients:

- 1 sweet potato
- 2 tablespoons olive oil
- 1/2 onion, chopped
- 1 carrot, peeled and chopped
- 2 garlic cloves, minced
- 1/2 teaspoon dried thyme
- 1 cup chopped kale
- Sea salt
- Freshly ground black pepper

Directions:

1. Pierce the sweet potato and microwave on high until soft, about 5 minutes. Remove from the microwave and cut into 1/4-inch cubes.
2. In a large nonstick sauté pan, heat the olive oil over medium-high heat. Add the onion and carrot and cook until softened, about 5 minutes. Attach the garlic and thyme until the garlic is fragrant, about 30 seconds.
3. Add the sweet potatoes and cook until the potatoes begin to brown, about 7 -minutes. Add the kale and cook just until it wilts, 1 to 2 minutes. Season with salt and pepper. Serve immediately.

Nutrition:

Calories: 125;

Fat: 9g;

Protein: 15g;

Carbohydrates: 35g;

Fiber: 17g;

Sugar: 18g;

Sodium: 310mg

Savory Oatmeal Porridge

Preparation Time: 5 minutes

Cooking time: 20 minutes

Servings: 4

Ingredients:

- 2 1/2 cups vegetable broth
- 2 1/2 cups milk
- 1/2 cup steel-cut oats
- 1 tablespoon faro
- 1/2 cup slivered almonds
- 1/4 cup nutritional yeast
- 2 cups old-fashioned rolled oats
- 1/2 teaspoon salt (optional)

Directions:

1. Take the broth and almond milk to a boil. Add the oats, faro, almond slivers, and nutritional yeast. Cook over medium-high heat for 20 minutes, stirring occasionally.
2. Add the rolled oats and cook for another 5 minutes, until creamy. Stir in the salt (if using).
3. Divide into 4 single-serving containers. Let cool before sealing the lids.

Nutrition:

Calories: 152;

Fat: 16g;

Protein: 35g;

Carbohydrates: 55g;

Fiber: 25g;

Sugar: 18g;

Sodium: 245mg

Pumpkin Steel-Cut Oats

Preparation Time: 15 minutes

Cooking time: 25 minutes

Servings: 4

Ingredients:

- 3 cups water
- 1 cup steel-cut oats
- 1/2 cup canned pumpkin purée
- 1/4 cup pumpkin seeds (pipits)
- 2 tablespoons maple syrup
- Pinch salt

Directions:

1. Whip and reduce the heat to low. Simmer until the oats are soft, 20 to 30 minutes, continuing to stir occasionally.
2. Stir in the pumpkin purée and continue cooking on low for 3 to 5 minutes longer. Stir in the pumpkin seeds and maple syrup, and season with the salt.
3. Divide the oatmeal into 4 single-serving containers. Let cool before sealing the lids.

Nutrition:

Calories: 132;

Fat: 19;

Protein: 4535g;

Carbohydrates: 75g;

Fiber: 73; g

Sugar: 15; g

Sodium: 345mg

Cinnamon and Spice Overnight Oats

Preparation Time: 15 minutes

Cooking time: 20 minutes

Servings: 3

Ingredients:

- 2.1/2 cups old-fashioned rolled oats
- 5 tablespoons pumpkin seeds (pipits)
- 5 tablespoons chopped pecans
- 5 cups unsweetened plant-based milk
- 21/2 teaspoons maple syrup or agave syrup
- 1/2 to 1 teaspoon salt
- 1/2 to 1 teaspoon ground cinnamon
- 1/2 to 1 teaspoon ground ginger

Directions:

1. Line up 5 wide-mouth pint jars. In each jar, combine 1/2 cup of oats, 1 tablespoon of pumpkin seeds, 1 tablespoon of pecans, 1 cup of plant-based milk, 1/2 teaspoon of maple syrup, 1 pinch of salt, 1 pinch of cinnamon, and 1 pinch of ginger.
2. Stir the ingredients in each jar. Close the jars tightly with lids. To serve, top with fresh fruit (if using).

Nutrition:

Calories: 124;

Fat: 1927

Protein: 35g;

Carbohydrates: 80;

Fiber: 65 g

Sugar: 18 g

Sodium: 276

Barley Breakfast Bowl

Preparation Time: 5 minutes

Cooking time: 15minutes

Servings: 4

Ingredients:

- 1.1/2 cups pearl barley
- 3.3/4 cups water
- Large pinch salt
- 1.1/2 cups dried cranberries
- 3 cups sweetened vanilla plant-based milk
- 2 tablespoons slivered almonds (optional)

Directions:

1. Put the barley, water, and salt. Bring to a boil.
2. Divide the barley into 6 jars or single-serving storage containers. Attached the 1/4 cup of dried cranberries to each. Pour 1/2 cup of plant-based milk into each. Attached the 1 teaspoon of slivered almonds (if using) to each. Close the jars tightly with lids.

Nutrition:

Calories: 109;

Fat: 15g;

Protein: 24g;

Carbohydrates: 32g;

Fiber: 8g;

Sugar: 1g;

Sodium: 466mg

Sweet Potato and Black Bean Hash

Preparation Time: 10 minutes

Cooking time: 20minutes

Servings: 6

Ingredients:

- 1 teaspoon extra-virgin olive oil or 3 teaspoons vegetable broth
- 1 large sweet yellow onion, diced
- 2 teaspoons minced garlic (about 2 cloves)
- 1 large sweet potato, unpeeled, diced into ¾-inch pieces
- 2 teaspoons ground cumin
- 1 teaspoon dried oregano
- 1 (14.5-ounce) can black beans, rinsed and drained
- 1/4 teaspoon salt
- 1/4 teaspoon freshly ground black pepper

Directions:

1. In large skillet over medium-high heat, heat the olive oil. Attach the onion and garlic and cook for 5 minutes, stirring frequently.
2. Add the sweet potatoes, cumin, and oregano. Stir and cook for another 5 minutes. Cover the skillet, reduce the heat to low, and cook for 15 minutes.
3. After 15 minutes, increase the heat to medium-high and stir in the black beans, salt (if using), and pepper. Cook for another 5 minutes.
4. Divide evenly among 6 single-serving containers. Let cool before sealing the lids.

Nutrition:

Calories: 209;

Fat: 12g;

Protein: 34g;

Carbohydrates: 22g;

Fiber: 8g;

Sugar: 1g;

Sodium: 466mg

Smoothie Breakfast Bowl

Preparation Time: 10 minutes

Cooking time: 20minutes

Servings: 4

Ingredients:

- 4 bananas, peeled
- 1 cup dragon fruit or fruit of choice
- 1 cup Baked Granola
- 2 cups fresh berries
- 1/2 cup slivered almonds
- 4 cups plant-based milk

Directions:

1. Open 4 quart-size, freezer-safe bags, and layer in the following order: 1 banana (halved or sliced) and 1/4 cup dragon fruit.
2. Into 4 small jelly jars, layer in the following order: 1/4 cup granola, 1/2 cup berries, and 2 tablespoons slivered almonds.
3. To serve, take a frozen bag of bananas and dragon fruit and transfer to a blender. Add 1 cup of plant-based milk, and blend until smooth. Pour into a bowl. Add the contents of 1 jar of granola, berries, and almonds over the top of the smoothie, and serve with a spoon.

Nutrition:

Calories: 109;

Fat: 12g;

Protein: 24g;

Carbohydrates: 24g;

Fiber: 8g;

Sugar: 5g;

Sodium: 366mg

Tortilla Breakfast Casserole

Preparation Time: 20 minutes

Cooking time: 20minutes

Servings: 4

Ingredients:

- 1 recipe Tofu-Spinach Scramble
- 1 (14-ounce) can black beans
- 1/4 cup nutritional yeast
- 2 teaspoons hot sauce
- 10 small corn tortillas
- 1/2 cup shredded vegan Cheddar or pepper Jack cheese, divided

Directions:

1. Preheat the oven to 350°F. Coat a 9-by-9-inch baking pan with cooking spray.
2. In a large bowl, combine the tofu scramble with the black beans, nutritional yeast, and hot sauce. Set aside.
3. In the bottom of the baking pan, place 5 corn tortillas. Spread half of the tofu and bean mixture over the tortillas. Spread 1/4 cup of cheese over the top. Layer the remaining 5 tortillas over the top of the cheese. Spread the reminder of the tofu and bean mixture over the tortillas. Spread the remaining 1/4 cup of cheese over the top.
4. Bake for 20 minutes.
5. Divide evenly among 6 single-serving containers. Let cool before sealing the lids.

Nutrition:

Calories: 132;

Fat: 10g;

Protein: 34g;

Carbohydrates: 54g;

Fiber: 9g;

Sugar: 4g;

Sodium: 254mg

Tofu-Spinach Scramble

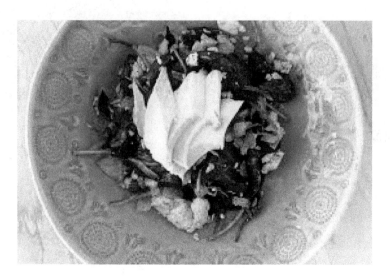

Preparation Time: 15 minutes

Cooking time: 20minutes

Servings: 5

Ingredients:

- 1 (14-ounce) package water-packed extra-firm tofu
- 1 teaspoon extra-virgin olive oil or 1/4 cup vegetable broth
- 1 small yellow onion, diced
- 3 teaspoons minced garlic (about 3 cloves)
- 3 large celery stalks, chopped
- 2 large carrots, peeled (optional) and chopped
- 1 teaspoon chili powder
- 1/2 teaspoon ground cumin
- 1/2 teaspoon ground turmeric
- 1/2 teaspoon salt (optional)
- 1/4 teaspoon freshly ground black pepper
- 5 cups loosely packed spinach

Directions:

1. Drain the tofu by placing it, wrapped in a paper towel, on a plate in the sink. Place a cutting board over the tofu, then set a heavy pot, can, or cookbook on the cutting board. Remove after 10 minutes. (Alternatively, use a tofu press.)

2. In a medium bowl, crumble the tofu with your hands or a potato masher.

3. Heat the olive oil. Add the onion, garlic, celery, and carrots, and sauté for 5 minutes, until the onion is softened.

4. Add the crumbled tofu, chili powder, cumin, turmeric, salt (if using), and pepper, and continue cooking for 7 to 8 more minutes, stirring frequently, until the tofu begins to brown.

5. Add the spinach and mix well. Cover and reduce the heat to medium. Steam the spinach for 3 minutes.

6. Divide evenly among 5 single-serving containers. Let cool before sealing the lids.

Nutrition:

Calories: 122;

Fat: 15g;

Protein: 14g;

Carbohydrates: 54g;

Fiber: 8g;

Sugar: 1g;

Sodium: 354mg

Savory Pancakes

Preparation Time: 10 minutes

Cooking time: 15minutes

Servings: 4

Ingredients:

- 1 cup whole-wheat flour
- 1 teaspoon garlic salt
- 1 teaspoon onion powder
- 1/2 teaspoon baking soda
- 1/4 teaspoon salt
- 1 cup lightly pressed, crumbled soft or firm tofu
- 1/2 cup unsweetened plant-based milk
- 1/4 cup lemon juice
- 2 tablespoons extra-virgin olive oil
- 1/2 cup finely chopped mushrooms
- 1/2 cup finely chopped onion
- 2 cups tightly packed greens (arugula, spinach, or baby kale work great)

Directions:

1. Attach the flour, garlic salt, onion powder, baking soda, and salt. Mix well. In a blender, combine the tofu, plant-based milk, lemon juice, and olive oil. Purée on high speed for 30 seconds.

2. Pour the contents of the blender into the bowl of dry ingredients and whisk until combined well. Fold in the mushrooms, onion, and greens.

Nutrition:

Calories: 132;

Fat: 10g;

Protein: 12g;

Carbohydrates: 44g;

Fiber: 9g;

Sodium: 254mg

Quinoa Breakfast Porridge

Preparation Time: 10 minutes

Cooking time: 5 minutes

Servings: 3

Ingredients:

- 1 cup dry quinoa
- 2 cups almond milk
- 1 tbsp. agave or maple syrup
- 1/2 tsp. vanilla
- 1/2 tsp. cinnamon
- 1 tablespoon ground flax meal

Directions:

1. Combine quinoa, almond milk, sugar, vanilla, and cinnamon in a little pot. Heat to the point of boiling and lessen to a stew.
2. Allow the quinoa to cook until the majority of the fluid is retained, and quinoa is fleecy (15-20 minutes). Blend in the flax meal. Blend in any extra toppers or include INS, and appreciate.

Nutrition:

Calories: 122;

Fat: 12g;

Protein: 12g;

Carbohydrates: 34g;

Fiber: 9g;

Sugar: 5g;

Sodium: 154mg

Grapes and Green Tea Smoothie

Preparation Time: 5 Minutes

Cooking Time: 0 Minutes

Servings: 2

Ingredients:

- ½ cup green tea
- ½ cup of green grapes
- 1 banana, peeled
- 1-inch piece of ginger
- ½ cup of ice cubes
- 2 cups baby spinach
- ½ of a medium apple, peeled, diced

Directions:

1. Place all the ingredients into the jar of a high-speed food processor or blender in the order stated in the ingredients list and then cover it with the lid.
2. Pulse for 1 minute until smooth, and then serve.

Nutrition:

Calories: 150 Cal;

Fat: 2.5 g;

Protein: 1 g;

Carbs: 36.5 g;

Fiber: 9 g

Mango and Kale Smoothie

Preparation Time: 5 Minutes

Cooking Time: 0 Minutes

Servings: 2

Ingredients:

- 2 cups oats milk, unsweetened
- 2 bananas, peeled
- ½ cup kale leaves
- 2 teaspoons coconut sugar
- 1 cup mango pieces
- 1 teaspoon vanilla extract, unsweetened

Directions:

1. Place all the ingredients into the jar of a high-speed food processor or blender in the order stated in the ingredients list and then cover it with the lid.
2. Pulse for 1 minute until smooth, and then serve.

Nutrition:

Calories: 281 Cal;

Fat: 3 g;

Protein: 6 g;

Carbs: 63 g;

Fiber: 16 g

Pomegranate Smoothie

Preparation Time: 5 Minutes

Cooking Time: 0 Minutes

Servings: 2

Ingredients:

- 2 cups almond milk, unsweetened
- 2 medium apples, cored, sliced
- 2 bananas, peeled
- 2 cups frozen raspberries
- 1 cup pomegranate seeds
- 4 teaspoons agave syrup

Directions:

1. Place all the ingredients into the jar of a high-speed food processor or blender in the order stated in the ingredients list and then cover it with the lid.
2. Pulse for 1 minute until smooth, and then serve.

Nutrition:

Calories: 141.5 Cal;

Fat: 1.1 g;

Protein: 4.1 g;

Carbs: 30.8 g;

Fiber: 2.4 g

Coconut Water Smoothie

Preparation Time: 5 Minutes

Cooking Time: 0 Minutes

Servings: 2

Ingredients:

- 2 cups of coconut water
- 1 large apple, peeled, cored, diced
- 1 cup of frozen mango pieces
- 2 teaspoons peanut butter
- 4 teaspoons coconut flakes

Directions:

1. Place all the ingredients into the jar of a high-speed food processor or blender in the order stated in the ingredients list and then cover it with the lid.
2. Pulse for 1 minute until smooth, and then serve.

Nutrition:

Calories: 113.4 Cal;

Fat: 0.3 g;

Protein: 0.6 g;

Carbs: 29 g;

Fiber: 2 g

Apple, Banana, and Berry Smoothie

Preparation Time: 5 Minutes

Cooking Time: 0 Minutes

Servings: 2

Ingredients:

- 2 cups almond milk, unsweetened

- 2 cups frozen strawberries

- 2 bananas, peeled

- 1 large apple, peeled, cored, diced

- 2 tablespoons peanut butter

Directions:

1. Place all the ingredients into the jar of a high-speed food processor or blender in the order stated in the ingredients list and then cover it with the lid.

2. Pulse for 1 minute until smooth, and then serve.

Nutrition:

Calories: 156.1 Cal;

Fat: 3.2 g;

Protein: 3 g;

Carbs: 17 g;

Fiber: 5.8 g

Berry Ginger Zing Smoothie

Preparation Time: 5 Minutes

Cooking Time: 0 Minutes

Servings: 2

Ingredients:

- 2 cups almond milk, unsweetened
- 1 cup frozen raspberries
- 1 cup of frozen strawberries
- 1 cup cauliflower florets
- 1-inch pieces of ginger

Directions:

1. Place all the ingredients into the jar of a high-speed food processor or blender in the order stated in the ingredients list and then cover it with the lid.
2. Pulse for 1 minute until smooth, and then serve.

Nutrition:

Calories: 300 Cal;

Fat: 8 g;

Protein: 8 g;

Carbs: 30 g;

Fiber: 9 g

Dragon Fruit Smoothie Bowl

Preparation Time: 5 Minutes

Cooking Time: 0 Minutes

Servings: 2

Ingredients:

For the Bowl:

- ½ cup coconut milk, unsweetened
- 2 bananas, peeled
- ½ cup frozen raspberries
- 7 ounces frozen dragon fruit
- 3 tablespoons vanilla protein powder

For the Toppings:

- 2 tablespoons coconut flakes
- 2 tablespoons hemp seeds

Directions:

1. Place all the ingredients for the bowl into the jar of a high-speed food processor or blender in the order stated in the ingredients list and then cover it with the lid.
2. Pulse for 1 minute until smooth, and then divide evenly between two bowls.
3. Sprinkle 1 tablespoon of coconut flakes and hemp seeds over the smoothie and then serve.

Nutrition:

Calories: 225 Cal;

Fat: 1.6 g;

Protein: 8.1 g;

Carbs: 48 g;

Fiber: 8.9 g

Chocolate Smoothie Bowl

Preparation Time: 5 Minutes

Cooking Time: 0 Minutes

Servings: 2

Ingredients:

For the Bowls:

- 2 cups almond milk, unsweetened
- 2 bananas, peeled
- 3 tablespoons cocoa powder
- 1 cup spinach leaves, fresh
- 2 tablespoons oat flour
- 4 Medjool dates, pitted
- 1/8 teaspoon salt
- 2 tablespoons vanilla protein powder
- 2 tablespoons peanut butter

For the Toppings:

- 2 tablespoons coconut flakes
- 2 tablespoons hemp seeds

Directions:

1. Place all the ingredients for the bowl into the jar of a high-speed food processor or blender in the order stated in the ingredients list and then cover it with the lid.
2. Pulse for 1 minute until smooth, and then divide evenly between two bowls.
3. Sprinkle 1 tablespoon of coconut flakes and hemp seeds over the smoothie and then serve.

Nutrition:

Calories: 382 Cal;

Fat: 14 g;

Protein: 22 g;

Carbs: 53 g;

Zucchini and Blueberry Smoothie

Preparation Time: 5 Minutes

Cooking Time: 0 Minutes

Servings: 2

Ingredients:

- 1 cup coconut milk, unsweetened
- 1 large celery stem
- 2 bananas, peeled
- ½ cup spinach leaves, fresh
- 1 cup frozen blueberries
- 2/3 cup sliced zucchini
- 1 tablespoon hemp seeds
- ½ teaspoon maca powder
- ¼ teaspoon ground cinnamon

Directions:

1. Place all the ingredients into the jar of a high-speed food processor or blender in the order stated in the ingredients list and then cover it with the lid.
2. Pulse for 1 minute until smooth, and then serve.

Nutrition:

Calories: 218 Cal;

Fat: 10.1 g;

Protein: 6.3 g;

Carbs: 31.8 g;

Fiber: 4.7 g

Hot Pink Beet Smoothie

Preparation Time: 5 Minutes

Cooking Time: 0 Minutes

Servings: 2

Ingredients:

- 2 cups almond milk, unsweetened
- 2 clementine, peeled
- 1 cup raspberries
- 1 banana, peeled
- 1 medium beet, peeled, chopped
- 2 tablespoons chia seeds
- 1/8 teaspoon sea salt
- ½ teaspoon vanilla extract, unsweetened
- 4 tablespoons almond butter

Directions:

1. Place all the ingredients into the jar of a high-speed food processor or blender in the order stated in the ingredients list and then cover it with the lid.
2. Pulse for 1 minute until smooth, and then serve.

Nutrition:

Calories: 260.8 Cal;

Fat: 1.3 g;

Protein: 13 g;

Carbs: 56 g;

Fiber: 9.3 g

Chickpea Flour Frittata

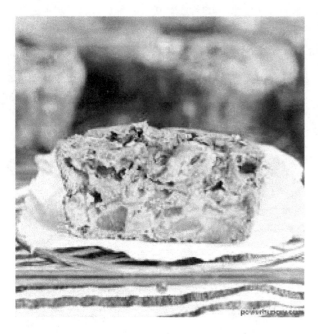

Preparation Time: 10 Minutes

Cooking Time: 50 Minutes

Servings: 6

Ingredients:

- 1 medium green bell pepper, cored, chopped

- 1 cup chopped greens

- 1 cup cauliflower florets, chopped

- ½ cup chopped broccoli florets

- ½ of a medium red onion, peeled, chopped

- ¼ teaspoon salt

- ½ cup chopped zucchini

For the Batter:

- ¼ cup cashew cream

- ½ cup chickpea flour

- ½ cup chopped cilantro

- ½ teaspoon salt

- ¼ teaspoon cayenne pepper

- ½ teaspoon dried dill

- ¼ teaspoon ground black pepper

- ¼ teaspoon dried thyme

- ½ teaspoon ground turmeric

- 1 tablespoon olive oil

- 1 ½ cup water

Directions:

1. Switch on the oven, then set it to 375 degrees F and let it preheat.

2. Take a 9-inch pie pan, grease it with oil, and then set aside until required.

3. Take a large bowl, place all the vegetables in it, sprinkle with salt and then toss until combined.

4. Prepare the batter and for this, add all of its ingredients in it except for thyme, dill, and cilantro and then pulse until combined and smooth.

5. Pour the batter over the vegetables, add dill, thyme, and cilantro, and then stir until combined.

6. Spoon the mixture into the prepared pan, spread evenly, and then bake for 45 to 50 minutes until done and inserted toothpick into frittata comes out clean.

7. When done, let the frittata rest for 10 minutes, cut it into slices, and then serve.

Nutrition:

Calories: 153 Cal;

Fat: 4 g;

Protein: 7 g;

Carbs: 20 g;

Fiber: 4 g

Potato Pancakes

Preparation Time: 10 Minutes

Cooking Time: 20 Minutes

Servings: 10

Ingredients:

- ½ cup white whole-wheat flour
- 3 large potatoes, grated
- ½ of a medium white onion, peeled, grated
- 1 jalapeno, minced
- 2 green onions, chopped
- 1 tablespoon minced garlic
- 1 teaspoon salt
- ¼ teaspoon baking powder
- ¼ teaspoon ground pepper
- 4 tablespoons olive oil

Directions:

1. Take a large bowl, place all the ingredients except for oil and then stir until well combined; stir in 1 to 2 tablespoons water if needed to mix the batter.

2. Take a large skillet pan, place it over medium-high heat, add 2 tablespoons of oil and then let it heat.

3. Scoop the pancake mixture in portions into the pan, shape each portion like a pancake and then cook for 5 to 7 minutes per side until pancakes turn golden brown and thoroughly cooked.

4. When done, transfer the pancakes to a plate, add more oil into the pan and then cook more pancakes in the same manner.

5. Serve straight away.

Nutrition:

Calories: 69 Cal;

Fat: 1 g;

Protein: 2 g;

Carbs: 12 g;

Chocolate Chip Pancakes

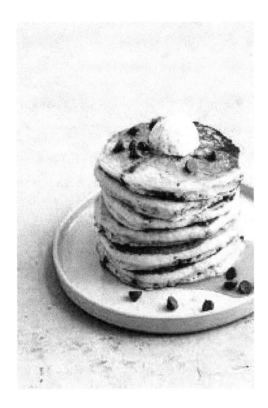

Preparation Time: 5 Minutes

Cooking Time: 10 Minutes

Servings: 6

Ingredients:

- 1 cup white whole-wheat flour
- ½ cup chocolate chips, vegan, unsweetened
- 1 tablespoon baking powder
- ¼ teaspoon salt
- 2 teaspoons coconut sugar
- ½ teaspoon vanilla extract, unsweetened

- 1 cup almond milk, unsweetened

- 2 tablespoons coconut butter, melted

- 2 tablespoons olive oil

Directions:

1. Take a large bowl, place all the ingredients except for oil and chocolate chips, and then stir until well combined.

2. Add chocolate chips, and then fold until just mixed.

3. Take a large skillet pan, place it over medium-high heat, add 1 tablespoon oil and then let it heat.

4. Scoop the pancake mixture in portions into the pan, shape each portion like a pancake and then cook for 5 to 7 minutes per side until pancakes turn golden brown and thoroughly cooked.

5. When done, transfer the pancakes to a plate, add more oil into the pan and then cook more pancakes in the same manner.

6. Serve straight away.

Nutrition:

Calories: 172 Cal;

Fat: 6 g;

Protein: 2.5 g;

Carbs: 28 g;

Fiber: 8 g

Turmeric Steel-Cut Oats

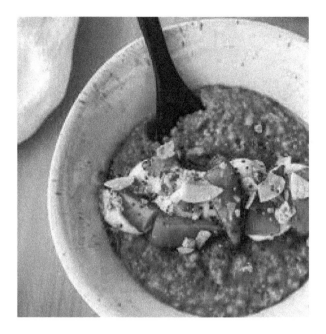

Preparation Time: 5 Minutes

Cooking Time: 10 Minutes

Servings: 2

Ingredients:

- ½ cup steel-cut oats

- 1/8 teaspoon salt

- 2 tablespoons maple syrup

- ½ teaspoon ground cinnamon

- 1/3 teaspoon turmeric powder

- ¼ teaspoon ground cardamom

- ¼ teaspoon olive oil

- ½ cups water

- 1 cup almond milk, unsweetened

For the Topping:

- 2 tablespoons pumpkin seeds

- 2 tablespoons chia seeds

Directions:

1. Take a medium saucepan, place it over medium heat, add oats, and then cook for 2 minutes until toasted.

2. Pour in the milk and water, stir until mixed, and then bring the oats to a boil.

3. Then switch heat to medium-low level, simmer the oats for 10 minutes, and add salt, maple syrup, and all spices.

4. Stir until combined, cook the oats for 7 minutes or more until cooked to the desired level and when done, let the oats rest for 15 minutes.

5. When done, divide oats evenly between two bowls, top with pumpkin seeds and chia seeds and then serve.

Nutrition:

Calories: 234 Cal;

Fat: 4 g;

Protein: 7 g;

Carbs: 41 g;

Fiber: 5 g

Vegetable Pancakes

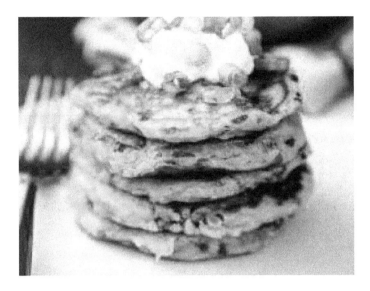

Preparation Time: 10 Minutes

Cooking Time: 20 Minutes

Servings: 10

Ingredients:

- 1/3 cup cooked and mashed sweet potato

- 2 cups grated carrots

- 1 cup chopped coriander

- 1 cup cooked spinach

- 2 ounces chickpea flour

- ½ teaspoon baking powder

- 1 ½ teaspoon salt

- 1 teaspoon ground turmeric

- 2 tablespoons olive oil

- ¾ cup of water

Directions:

1. Take a large bowl, place chickpea flour in it, add turmeric powder, baking powder, and salt, and then stir until combined.

2. Whisk in the water until combined, stir in sweet potatoes until well mixed and then add carrots, spinach, and coriander until well combined.

3. Take a large skillet pan, place it over medium-high heat, add 1 tablespoon oil and then let it heat.

4. Scoop the pancake mixture in portions into the pan, shape each portion like a pancake and then cook for 3 to 5 minutes per side until pancakes turn golden brown and thoroughly cooked.

5. When done, transfer the pancakes to a plate, add more oil into the pan and then cook more pancakes in the same manner.

6. Serve straight away.

Nutrition:

Calories: 74 Cal;

Fat: 0.3 g;

Protein: 3 g;

Carbs: 16 g;

Fiber: 2.7 g

Banana and Chia Pudding

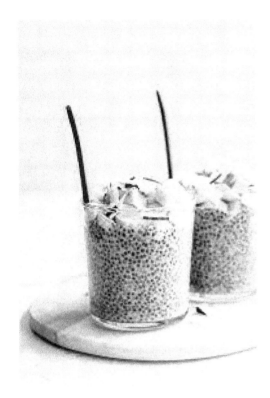

Preparation Time: 25 Minutes

Cooking Time: 12 Minutes

Servings: 2

Ingredients:

For the Pudding:

- 2 bananas, peeled

- 4 tablespoons chia seeds

- 2 tablespoons coconut sugar

- ½ teaspoon pumpkin pie spice

- 1/8 teaspoon sea salt

- ½ cup almond milk, unsweetened

For the Bananas:

- 2 bananas, peeled, sliced

- 2 tablespoons coconut flakes

- 1/8 teaspoon ground cinnamon

- 2 tablespoons coconut sugar

- ¼ cup chopped walnuts

- 2 tablespoons almond milk, unsweetened

Directions:

1. Prepare the pudding and for this, place all of its ingredients in a blender except for chia seeds and then pulse until smooth.

2. Pour the mixture into a medium saucepan, place it over medium heat, bring the mixture to a boil and then remove the pan from heat.

3. Add chia seeds into the hot banana mixture, stir until mixed, and then let it sit for 5 minutes.

4. Whisk the pudding and then let it chill for 15 minutes in the refrigerator.

5. Meanwhile, prepare the caramelized bananas and for this, take a medium skillet pan, and place it over medium heat.

6. Add banana slices, sprinkle with salt, sugar, and nutmeg, drizzle with milk and then cook for 5 minutes until mixture has thickened.

7. Assemble the pudding and for this, divide the pudding evenly between two bowls, top with banana slices, sprinkle with walnuts, and then serve.

Nutrition:

Calories: 495 Cal;

Fat: 21 g;

Protein: 9 g;

Carbs: 76 g;

Fiber: 14 g

Tofu Scramble

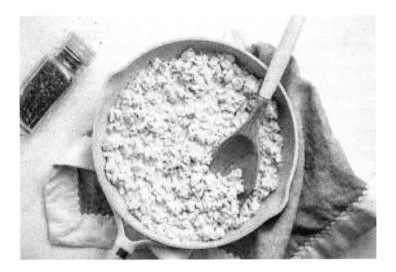

Preparation Time: 5 Minutes

Cooking Time: 15 Minutes

Servings: 3

Ingredients:

- 12 ounces tofu, extra-firm, pressed, drained
- ½ of a medium red onion, peeled, sliced
- 1 cup baby greens mix
- 1 medium red bell pepper, cored, sliced
- ½ teaspoon garlic powder
- 1 teaspoon salt
- ½ teaspoon ground black pepper
- ¼ teaspoon turmeric powder
- ¼ teaspoon ground cumin
- 4 tablespoons olive oil, divided

Directions:

1. Take a large bowl, place tofu in it, and then break it into bite-size pieces.

2. Add salt, black pepper, turmeric, and 2 tablespoons of oil, and then stir until mixed.

3. Take a medium skillet pan, place it over medium heat, add garlic powder and cumin and then cook for 1 minute until fragrant.

4. Add tofu mixture, stir until mixed, switch heat to medium-high level, and then cook for 5 minutes until tofu turn golden brown.

5. When done, divide tofu evenly between three plates, keep it warm, and then set aside until required.

6. Return the skillet pan over medium-high heat, add remaining oil and let it heat until hot.

7. Add onion and bell peppers, cook for 5 to 7 minutes or until beginning to brown, and then season with a pinch of salt.

8. Add baby greens, toss until mixed, and then cook for 30 seconds until leaves begin to wilts.

9. Add vegetables evenly to the plates to scrambled tofu and then serve.

Nutrition:

Calories: 304 Cal;

Fat: 25.6 g;

Protein: 14.2 g;

Carbs: 6.6 g;

Fiber: 2.6 g

Pumpkin Spice Oatmeal

Preparation Time: 5 Minutes

Cooking Time: 8 Minutes

Servings: 2

Ingredients:

- ¼ cup Medjool dates, pitted, chopped
- 2/3 cup rolled oats
- 1 tablespoon maple syrup
- ½ teaspoon pumpkin pie spice
- ½ teaspoon vanilla extract, unsweetened
- 1/3 cup pumpkin puree
- 2 tablespoons chopped pecans
- 1 cup almond milk, unsweetened

Directions:

1. Take a medium pot, place it over medium heat, and then add all the ingredients except for pecans and maple syrup.
2. Stir all the ingredients until combined, and then cook for 5 minutes until the oatmeal has absorbed all the liquid and thickened to the desired level.
3. When done, divide oatmeal evenly between two bowls, top with pecans, drizzle with maple syrup and then serve.

Nutrition:

Calories: 175 Cal;

Fat: 3.2 g;

Protein: 5.8 g;

Carbs: 33 g;

Fiber: 6.1 g

Peanut Butter Bites

Preparation Time: 10 Minutes

Cooking Time: 0 Minutes

Servings: 5

Ingredients:

- 1 cup rolled oats

- 12 Medjool dates, pitted

- ½ cup peanut butter, sugar-free

Directions:

1. Plug in a blender or a food processor, add all the ingredients in its jar, and then cover with the lid.

2. Pulse for 5 minutes until well combined, and then tip the mixture into a shallow dish.

3. Shape the mixture into 20 balls, 1 tablespoon of mixture per ball, and then serve.

Nutrition:

Calories: 103.1 Cal;

Fat: 4.3 g;

Protein: 2.3 g;

Carbs: 15.4 g;

Fiber: 0.8 g

Maple and Cinnamon Overnight Oats

Preparation Time: 10 Minutes

Cooking Time: 0 Minutes

Servings: 4

Ingredients:

- 2 cups rolled oats
- ¼ cup chopped pecans
- ¾ teaspoon ground cinnamon
- 1 teaspoon vanilla extract, unsweetened
- 3 tablespoons coconut sugar
- 3 tablespoons maple syrup
- 2 cups almond milk, unsweetened

Directions:

1. Take four mason jars, and then add ½ cup oats, ¼ teaspoon vanilla, and ½ cup milk.
2. Take a small bowl, add maple syrup, cinnamon, and sugar, stir until mixed, add this mixture into the oats mixture and then stir until combined.
3. Cover the jars with the lid and then let them rest in the refrigerator for a minimum of 2 hours or more until thickened.
4. When ready to eat, top the oats with pecans, sprinkle with cinnamon, drizzle with maple syrup and then serve.

Nutrition:

Calories: 292 Cal;

Fat: 9 g;

Protein: 7 g;

Carbs: 48 g;

Fiber: 6 g

Coconut Blackberry Breakfast Bowl

Preparation time: 15 minutes

Cooking time: 2 minutes

Servings: 2

Ingredients:

- 2 tbsp chia seeds
- ¼ cup coconut flakes
- 1 cup spinach
- ¼ cup of water
- 3 tbsp ground flaxseed
- 1 cup unsweetened coconut milk
- 1 cup blackberries

Directions:

1. Add blackberries, flaxseed, spinach, and coconut milk into the blender and blend until smooth. Fry coconut flakes in the pan for 1-2 minutes.
2. Pour berry mixture into the serving bowls and sprinkle coconut flakes and chia seeds on top. Serve immediately and enjoy.

Nutrition:

Calories 182

Fat 11.4 g

Carbohydrates 14.5 g

Protein 5.3 g

Cinnamon Coconut Pancake

Preparation time: 15 minutes

Cooking time: 10 minutes

Servings: 1

Ingredients:

- 1/2 cup almond milk
- 1/4 cup coconut flour
- 2 tbsp egg replacer
- 8 tbsp water
- 1 packet stevia
- 1/8 tsp cinnamon
- 1/2 tsp baking powder
- 1 tsp vanilla extract
- 1/8 tsp salt

Directions:

1. Mix egg replacer and 8 tablespoons of water in a small bowl. Add all ingredients into the mixing bowl and stir until combined.
2. Spray pan with cooking spray and heat over medium heat. Pour the desired amount of batter onto the hot pan and cook until lightly golden brown. Flip pancake and cook within a few minutes more. Serve and enjoy.

Nutrition:

Calories 110

Fat 4.3 g

Carbohydrates 10.9 g

Protein 7 g

Flax Almond Muffins

Preparation time: 15 minutes

Cooking time: 0 minutes

Servings: 6

Ingredients:

- 1 tsp cinnamon
- 2 tbsp coconut flour
- 20 drops liquid stevia
- 1/4 cup water
- 1/4 tsp vanilla extract
- 1/4 tsp baking soda
- 1/2 tsp baking powder
- 1/4 cup almond flour
- 1/2 cup ground flax
- 2 tbsp ground chia

Directions:

1. Warm oven to 350 F. Spray a muffin tray with cooking spray and set aside. Put 6 tablespoons of water and ground chia in a small bowl. Mix well and set aside.
2. In a mixing bowl, add ground flax, baking soda, baking powder, cinnamon, coconut flour, and almond flour and mix well.
3. Add chia seed mixture, vanilla, water, and liquid stevia and stir well to combine. Pour mixture into the prepared muffin tray and bake in preheated oven for 35 minutes. Serve and enjoy.

Nutrition:

Calories 92

Fat 6.3 g

Carbohydrates 6.9 g

Protein 3.7 g

Grain-Free Overnight Oats

Preparation time: 15 minutes

Cooking time: 0 minutes

Servings: 1

Ingredients:

- 2/3 cup unsweetened coconut milk
- 2 tsp chia seeds
- 2 tbsp vanilla protein powder
- ½ tbsp coconut flour
- 3 tbsp hemp hearts

Directions:

1. Add all ingredients into the glass jar and stir to combine. Close jar with lid and place in the refrigerator overnight. Top with fresh berries and serve.

Nutrition:

Calories 378

Fat 22.5 g

Carbohydrates 15 g

Protein 27 g

Apple Avocado Coconut Smoothie

Preparation time: 5 minutes

Cooking time: 0 minutes

Servings: 2

Ingredients:

- 1 tsp coconut oil
- 1 tbsp collagen powder
- 1 tbsp fresh lime juice
- ½ cup unsweetened coconut milk
- ¼ apple, slice
- 1 avocado

Directions:

1. Add all fixings into the blender and blend until smooth and creamy. Serve and enjoy.

Nutrition:

Calories 262

Fat 23.9 g

Carbohydrates 13.6 g

Protein 2 g

Chia Cinnamon Smoothie

Preparation time: 5 minutes

Cooking time: 0 minutes

Servings: 1

Ingredients:

- 2 scoops of vanilla protein powder
- 1 tbsp chia seeds
- ½ tsp cinnamon
- 1 tbsp coconut oil
- ½ cup of water
- ½ cup unsweetened coconut milk

Directions:

1. Add all fixings into the blender and blend until smooth and creamy. Serve immediately and enjoy.

Nutrition:

Calories 397

Fat 23.9 g

Carbohydrates 13.4 g

Protein 31.6 g

Strawberry Chia Matcha Pudding

Preparation time: 4 hours & 15 minutes

Cooking time: 0 minutes

Servings: 1

Ingredients:

- 5 drops liquid stevia
- 2 strawberries, diced
- 1 ½ tbsp chia seeds
- ¾ cup unsweetened coconut milk
- ½ tsp matcha powder

Directions:

1. Add all ingredients except strawberries into the glass jar and mix well. Close jar with lid and place in the refrigerator for 4 hours.
2. Add strawberries into the pudding and mix well. Serve and enjoy.

Nutrition:

Calories 93

Fat 6.5 g

Carbohydrates 5.6 g

Protein 2.5 g

Spinach Green Smoothie

Preparation time: 5 minutes

Cooking time: 0 minutes

Servings: 1

Ingredients:

- 1 cup ice cube
- 2/3 cup water
- ½ cup unsweetened almond milk
- 5 drops liquid stevia
- ½ tsp matcha powder
- 1 tsp vanilla extract
- 1 tbsp MCT oil
- ½ avocado
- 2/3 cup spinach

Directions:

1. Add all fixings into the blender and blend until smooth and creamy. Serve immediately and enjoy.

Nutrition:

Calories 167

Fat 18.3 g

Carbohydrates 3.8 g

Protein 1.6 g

Chapter 3.   Lunch

Tangy Broccoli Salad

Preparation time: 15 minutes

Cooking time: 0 minutes

Servings: 4

Ingredients:

- 2 heads broccoli, stems, and florets chopped (about 5 cups)
- 3 scallions, thinly sliced
- ½ cup carrots, grated
- ¼ cup hemp hearts
- 2 tablespoons tahini
- 2 tablespoons apple cider vinegar
- 2 tablespoons water
- 2 teaspoons maple syrup
- 1 garlic clove
- ¼ teaspoon salt
- Freshly ground black pepper

Directions:

1. Place the broccoli, scallions, carrots, and hemp hearts in a large bowl. Whisk the tahini, vinegar, water, maple syrup, garlic, and salt in a measuring cup or small bowl. Add as much pepper as you'd like.

2. Put the dressing over the salad and mix until everything is well combined.

Nutrition:

Calories: 189

Fat: 11g

Carbohydrate: 15g

Protein: 10g

Summer Rolls with Peanut Sauce

Preparation time: 15 minutes

Cooking time: 0 minutes

Servings: 4-6

Ingredients:

- 6 to 8 Vietnamese/Thai round rice paper wraps

- 1 (13-ounce) package organic, extra-firm smoked or plain tofu, drained, cut into long, thin slices

- 1 cucumber, cored, cut into matchsticks (about 1 cup)

- 1 cup carrot, cut into matchsticks

- 1 cup mung bean or soybean sprouts

- 4 to 6 cups of spinach

- 12 to 16 basil leaves

- 3 to 4 mint sprigs

- Sweet Peanut Dressing

Directions:

1. Place the rice paper wrap under running water or in a large bowl of water for a moment, then set it on a plate or cutting board to absorb the water for 30 seconds. The wrap should be transparent and pliable.

2. Place your desired amount of filling on each wrap, being careful not to overfill because they will be hard to close.

3. Tightly fold the bottom of the wraps over the ingredients, and then fold in each side. Continue rolling each wrap onto itself to form the rolls. Enjoy your rolls dipped in sweet peanut dressing.

Nutrition:

Calories: 216

Fat: 6g

Carbohydrate: 32g

Protein: 13g

Cheesy White Bean Cauliflower Soup

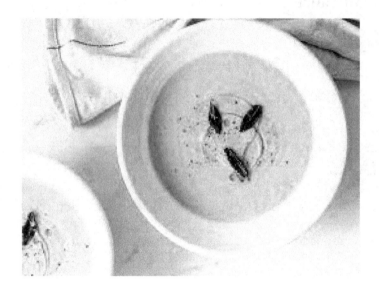

Preparation time: 15 minutes

Cooking time: 35 minutes

Servings: 6

Ingredients:

- 1 tablespoon olive oil

- 1 onion, chopped

- 2 celery stalks, chopped

- 2 carrots, chopped

- 3 garlic cloves, minced

- 1 teaspoon turmeric

- 1 head cauliflower, chopped into florets (about 5 cups)

- 4 cups vegetable broth

- 1 cup unsweetened nondairy milk

- ¼ cup nutritional yeast

- 1 teaspoon onion powder

- ½ teaspoon salt

- Juice of ½ lemon

- 2 (14-ounce) cans of white navy or cannellini beans, drained and rinsed

- Freshly ground black pepper

Directions:

1. In a large stockpot, warm the oil over medium heat. Add the onion, celery, and carrots. Cook until the onions become slightly translucent, within 5 minutes. Add the garlic and turmeric and cook for 1 minute more.

2. Add the cauliflower and broth, cover, and bring to a boil. Once boiling, reduce the heat and simmer, covered, until the cauliflower has softened, about 10 minutes. Pour in the milk, yeast, onion powder, and salt, and stir it.

3. Remove the pot and either use an immersion blender to purée the soup or transfer it to a blender and process it until smooth.

4. Once a smooth consistency is reached, return the soup to heat and add the lemon juice and beans. Stir and taste it; add extra salt and black pepper, if desired. Enjoy this soup with hot sauce.

Nutrition:

Calories: 238

Fat: 4g

Carbohydrate: 37g

Protein: 15g

Split Pea Soup

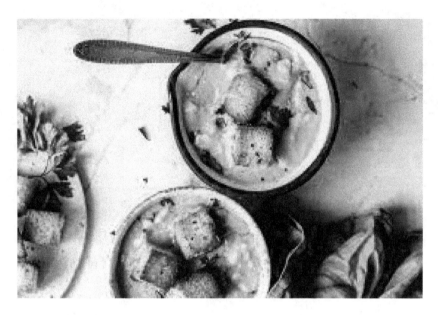

Preparation time: 15 minutes

Cooking time: 60 minutes

Servings: 6

Ingredients:

- 2 tablespoons olive oil

- 1 medium onion, coarsely chopped

- 2 carrots, coarsely chopped

- 2 celery stalks, coarsely chopped

- Pinch + 2 teaspoons salt, divided

- 2 cups yellow split peas, rinsed & drained

- 8 cups of water

- 1 bay leaf

- 1 teaspoon paprika

- Freshly ground black pepper

- 6 cups spinach, chopped

- 2 vegan sausages or spicy store-bought, chopped (optional)

Directions:

1. In a large stockpot, warm the oil over medium heat. Add the onion, carrots, celery, and a pinch of salt and cook until the onions start to soften.

2. Add the split peas, water, bay leaf, paprika, remaining 2 teaspoons of salt, and pepper. Bring to a boil.

3. Adjust the heat to low, then simmer, occasionally stirring, until the split peas are soft and the soup is thick about 50 minutes.

4. Remove and discard the bay leaf. Stir in the spinach and sausage (if using) and cook for a couple of minutes more—taste, adjust seasonings with salt and pepper.

Nutrition:

Calories: 362

Fat: 10g

Carbohydrate: 46g

Protein: 25g

Quinoa & Chickpea Tabbouleh

Preparation time: 25 minutes

Cooking time: 0 minutes

Servings: 6

Ingredients:

- 1 cup quinoa, cooked
- 1 cup tomato, chopped
- 1 cup cucumber, chopped
- 1 cup scallions, chopped
- 1 cup fresh parsley, chopped
- 1 (14-ounce) can chickpeas, drained and rinsed
- 2 garlic cloves, minced
- ¼ cup chopped mint/1 tablespoon dried mint
- 2 tablespoons olive oil
- Juice of 1 lemon
- ½ teaspoon salt
- Freshly ground black pepper

Directions:

1. Mix the quinoa, tomato, cucumber, scallions, parsley, chickpeas, garlic, and mint in a large bowl.

2. Pour the olive oil plus lemon juice over the quinoa mixture, and then stir in the salt and as much pepper as you'd like. Stir until everything is well combined. Enjoy immediately.

Nutrition:

Calories: 170

Fat: 6g

Carbohydrate: 25g

Protein: 6g

Cauliflower Caesar Salad with Chickpea Croutons

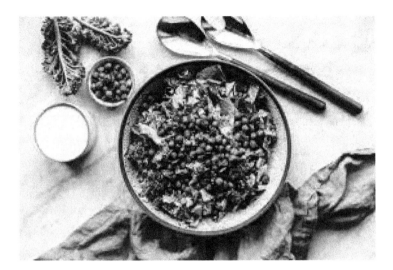

Preparation time: 15 minutes

Cooking time: 40 minutes

Servings: 4

Ingredients:

- 1 head cauliflower, chopped (about 8 cups)

- 3 tablespoons oil, divided

- A few pinches salt + ¼ teaspoon, divided

- 1 (14-ounce) can chickpeas, drained and rinsed

- 1 teaspoons oregano

- ¼ teaspoon garlic powder

- ¼ teaspoon onion powder

- 2 heads romaine lettuce, chopped

- Tofu Caesar Dressing

Directions:

1. Preheat the oven to 450°F. Prepare two baking sheets lined using parchment paper or silicone liners.

2. Mix the cauliflower, 2 tablespoons of olive oil, and a few big pinches of salt in a large bowl. Mix to ensure the cauliflower is well coated with oil. Spread the cauliflower out evenly on one of the baking sheets.

3. In a medium bowl, combine the chickpeas, the remaining 1 tablespoon of olive oil, oregano, garlic powder, onion powder, and the remaining ¼ teaspoon of salt. Spread the chickpeas out evenly on the other baking sheet.

4. Place the sheets in the oven and bake for 20 minutes; then give the sheet with the chickpeas a bit of a shake to ensure they aren't sticking or burning. Continue baking for 20 minutes more or until the cauliflower is soft and the chickpeas are crunchy.

5. To serve, divide the lettuce among 4 bowls and top each with even portions of the cauliflower, chickpeas, and about ¼ cup of Caesar dressing.

Nutrition:

Calories: 365

Fat: 20g

Carbohydrate: 37g

Protein: 16g

Vegetable Rose Potato

Preparation time: 15 minutes

Cooking time: 20 minutes

Servings: 4

Ingredients:

- 4 red rose potatoes

- 6 leaves Lacinato kale, stemmed, chopped

- 2 tablespoons olive oil

- 1 onion, chopped

- 1 green bell pepper, diced

- 1 teaspoon smoked paprika

- 1 teaspoon seasoning, salt-free

- Ground pepper, salt, to taste

Directions:

1. Microwave your potatoes until done but still firm. Finely chop them when cool.

2. Preheat oil in a skillet over medium heat. Sauté onions until translucent. Add potatoes and bell pepper and sauté, stirring constantly, over medium-high heat until golden brown.

3. Stir in the kale and seasoning, then cook, stirring constantly until the mixture is a bit browned. Occasionally add water to prevent sticking if necessary. Sprinkle with pepper and salt to taste. Serve hot.

Nutrition:

Calories 337

Fat 7.4 g

Carbs 63 g

Protein 8 g

Rice Arugula Salad

Preparation time: 15 minutes

Cooking time: 8 minutes

Servings: 2

Ingredients:

- 1 cup wild rice, cooked
- 1 handful arugula, washed
- ¾ cup almonds
- 6 sun-dried tomatoes in oil, chopped
- 3 tablespoons olive oil
- 1 onion
- Pepper and salt, to taste

Directions:

1. Put your frying pan over low heat and roast the almonds for 3 minutes. Transfer to a salad bowl.

2. Sauté onions in 1/3 olive oil for 3 minutes on low heat. Add dried tomatoes and cook for about 2 minutes. Transfer to a bowl.

3. Add the remaining olive oil to the pan and fry the bread until crunchy. Sprinkle with pepper and salt. Set aside.

4. Add arugula to the bowl containing sautéed tomato mixture. Add wild rice and toss to combine. Season with pepper, salt.

Nutrition:

Calories 688

Fat 37.7 g

Carbs 56 g

Protein 19 g

Tomato Salad

Preparation time: 15 minutes

Cooking time: 0 minutes

Servings: 4

Ingredients:

- 1 head romaine lettuce, washed, chopped
- 1 avocado, sliced
- 24 cherry tomatoes
- ½ cup cilantro, chopped
- Fresh lime juice, for dressing

Directions:

1. Divide all the ingredients between 4 plates and drizzle with lime juice dressing. Toss well to combine. Enjoy immediately.

Nutrition:

Calories 203

Fat 16.2 g

Carbs 12 g

Protein 6 g

Kale Apple Roasted Root Vegetable Salad

Preparation time: 15 minutes

Cooking time: 25 minutes

Servings: 6

Ingredients:

- 1 ½ cups parsnips, turnips and red rose potatoes, diced

- 8 cups kale, chopped

- ½ cup apple chunks

- 2 tablespoon apple cider vinegar

- ½ teaspoon cinnamon

- ½ teaspoon turmeric

- 4 tablespoons olive oil, divided

- Salt and pepper, to taste

Directions:

1. Place a skillet over medium heat. Add vinegar, apple, cinnamon, turmeric and salt. Bring the mixture to a boil and set aside.

2. Preheat the oven to 350 F. Preheat oil in a cast iron pan over medium heat. Add parsnips, turnips and red rose potatoes and cook for about 5 minutes.

3. Transfer to the oven and roast for about 10 minutes. Place a skillet over medium heat. Add the remaining olive oil. To the skillet add the kale and apples and cook for about 4 minutes

4. Add the parsnips, turnips, red rose potatoes and vinegar mixture to the skillet. Cook for about 5 minutes. Add salt and pepper to taste. Serve while hot and enjoy!

Nutrition:

Calories 128

Fat 16 g

Carbs 32 g

Protein 3 g

Rice Arugula Salad with Sesame Garlic Dressing

Preparation time: 15 minutes

Cooking time: 0 minutes

Servings: 4

Ingredients:

- 1 cup wild rice, cooked
- 1/8 teaspoon cumin
- ½ bunch arugula, chopped
- 2 tablespoons parsley, chopped
- 2 tablespoons basil, chopped
- Salt and black pepper, to taste

For the dressing:

- 1 head garlic, roasted and peeled
- ½ cup apple juice
- ¼ cup lemon juice
- ¼ cup tahini
- ¼ cup virgin olive oil
- Salt, to taste

Directions:

1. Add the dressing ingredients to a blender and blend until the mixture is creamy and smooth. Set aside.

2. Place a stockpot over medium high heat. Season rice with cumin and salt. Pour half of the dressing on top and mix well. Set aside to chill for about 10 minutes.

3. To the bowl add arugula, parsley, basil, olives, salt and pepper. Serve and enjoy!

Nutrition:

Calories 447

Fat 44.4 g

Carbs 43 g

Protein 19 g

Roasted Lemon Asparagus Watercress Salad

Preparation time: 15 minutes

Cooking time: 5 minutes

Servings: 4

Ingredients:

- 2 cups asparagus, ends trimmed
- 2 cups watercress
- 2 cups baby spinach
- 1 lemon, sliced, seeded
- 1 onion, sliced
- 1/8 teaspoon cayenne
- 2 tablespoons olive oil
- Salt and pepper, to taste

Directions:

1. Preheat 1 tablespoon oil in a skillet over medium heat. Add the asparagus and cook for about 5 minutes. Set aside. Return the skillet to medium low heat. Add the remaining olive oil.

2. Add onion and lemon slices and cook for about 5 minutes. Remove from heat and season with salt, cayenne and pepper.

3. Add the baby spinach in a large bowl. Add cooked onion and lemon slices on top. Finally add the asparagus. Serve and enjoy!

Nutrition:

Calories 129

Fat 7 g

Carbs 11 g

Protein 5 g

Pumpkin and Brussels Sprouts Mix

Preparation time: 15 minutes

Cooking time: 35-40 minutes

Servings: 8

Ingredients:

- 1 lb. Brussels sprouts, halved

- 1 pumpkin, peeled, cubed

- 4 garlic cloves, sliced

- 2 tablespoons fresh parsley, chopped

- 2 tablespoons balsamic vinegar

- 1/3 cup olive oil

- Salt, pepper, to taste

Directions:

1. Warm oven to 400 degrees F. Prepare a baking dish and coat with cooking spray. Mix sprouts, pumpkin and garlic in a bowl. Add oil and toss well to coat the vegetables.

2. Transfer to the baking dish and cook for 35-40 minutes. Stir once halfway. Serve topped with parsley.

Nutrition:

Calories 152

Fat 9 g

Carbohydrate 17 g

Protein 4 g

Almond and Tomato Salad

Preparation time: 15 minutes

Cooking time: 10 minutes

Servings: 4

Ingredients:

- 1 cup arugula/ rocket

- 7 oz fresh tomatoes, sliced or chopped

- 2 teaspoons olive oil

- 2 cups kale

- 1/2 cup almonds

Directions:

1. Put oil into your pan and heat it on a medium heat. Add tomatoes into the pan and fry for about 10 minutes. Once cooked, allow it to cool. Combine all salad ingredients in a bowl and serve.

Nutrition:

Calories 355

Fat 19.1 g

Carbohydrate 8.3 g

Protein 33 g

Strawberry Spinach Salad

Preparation time: 15 minutes

Cooking time: 0 minutes

Servings: 4

Ingredients:

- 5 cups baby spinach

- 2 cups strawberries, sliced

- 2 tablespoons lemon juice

- 1/2 teaspoon Dijon mustard

- 1/4 cup olive oil

- 3/4 cup toasted almonds, chopped

- 1/4 red onion, sliced

- Salt, pepper, to taste

Directions:

1. Take a large bowl and mix Dijon mustard with lemon juice in it, and slowly add olive oil and combine. Season the mixture with black pepper and salt.

2. Now, mix strawberries, half cup of almonds, and sliced onion in a bowl. Pour the dressing on top and toss to combine. Serve the salad topped with almonds and vegan cheese.

Nutrition:

Calories 116

Fat 3 g

Carbs 13 g

Protein 6 g

Apple Spinach Salad

Preparation time: 15 minutes

Cooking time: 0 minutes

Servings: 4

Ingredients:

- 5 ounces fresh spinach
- 1/4 red onion, sliced
- 1 apple, sliced
- 1/4 cup sliced toasted almonds

For the Dressing:

- 3 tablespoons red wine vinegar
- 1/3 cup olive oil
- 1 minced garlic clove
- 2 teaspoons Dijon mustard
- Salt, pepper, to taste

Directions:

1. Combine red wine vinegar, olive oil, garlic, and Dijon mustard in a bowl. Season with black pepper and salt.

2. In a separate bowl mix fresh spinach, apple, onion, toasted almonds. Pour the dressing on top and toss to combine. Serve

Nutrition:

Calories 232

Fat 20.8 g

Carbs 10 g

Protein 3 g

Kale Power Salad

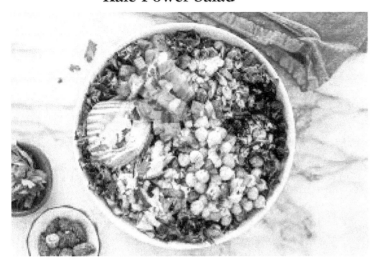

Preparation time: 15 minutes

Cooking time: 40 minutes

Servings: 2

Ingredients:

- 1 bunch kale, ribs removed and chopped
- 1/2 cup quinoa
- 1 tablespoon olive oil
- 1/2 lime, juiced
- ½ teaspoon salt
- 1 tablespoon olive oil
- 1 red rose potato, cut into small cubes
- 1 teaspoon ground cumin
- 3/4 teaspoons salt
- 1/2 teaspoon smoked paprika
- 1 lime, juiced
- 1 avocado, sliced into long strips
- 1 tablespoon olive oil

- 1 tablespoon cilantro leaves

- 1 jalapeno, deseeded, membranes removed and chopped

- salt

- ¼ cup pepitas

Directions:

1. Rinse quinoa in a running water for 2 minutes. Mix 2 cups water and rinsed quinoa in a pot, reduce heat to simmer and cook for 15 minutes.

2. Remove quinoa from heat and let rest, covered, for 5 minutes. Uncover pot, drain excess water and fluff quinoa with a fork. Let cool.

3. Warm-up olive oil in a pan over medium heat. Add chopped red rose potatoes and toss. Add smoked paprika, cumin and salt. Mix to combine.

4. Add ¼ cup water once pan is sizzling. Cover the pan then adjust heat to low. Cook for 10 minutes, stirring occasionally. Uncover pan, raise heat to medium and cook for 7 minutes. Set aside to cool.

5. Transfer kale to a bowl and add salt to it and massage with hands. Scrunch handfuls of kale in your hands. Repeat until kale is darker in color.

6. Mix 2 tablespoons olive oil, ½ teaspoon salt and 1 lime juice in a bowl. Add over the kale and toss to coat.

7. Add 2 avocados, 2 lime juices, 2 tablespoons olive oil, jalapeno, cilantro leaves and salt in a blender. Blend well and season the avocado sauce.

8. Toast pepitas in a skillet over medium low heat for 5 minutes, stirring frequently. Add quinoa to the kale bowl and toss to combine well.

9. Divide kale and quinoa mixture into 4 bowls. Top with red rose potatoes, avocado sauce, and pepitas. Enjoy!

Nutrition:

Calories 250

Fat 11 g

Carbs 25 g

Protein 9 g

Falafel Kale Salad with Tahini Dressing

Preparation time: 15 minutes

Cooking time: 0 minutes

Servings: 4

Ingredients:

- 12 balls Vegan Falafels
- 6 cups kale, chopped
- 1/2 red onion, thinly sliced
- 2 slices pita bread, cut in squares
- 1 jalapeño, chopped
- Tahini Dressing
- 1-2 lemons, juiced

Directions:

1. In a mixing bowl, combine kale and lemon juice and toss well to mix. Place into the refrigerator. Divide kale among four bowls.

2. Top with three Falafel balls, red onion, jalapeño and pita slices. Top with tahini dressing and serve.

Nutrition:

Calories 178

Fat 2.8 g

Carbs 16 g

Protein 4 g

Fig and Kale Salad

Preparation time: 15 minutes

Cooking time: 0 minutes

Servings: 2

Ingredients:

- 1 ripe avocado
- 2 tablespoons lemon juice
- 3 ½ oz kale, packed, stems removed and cut into large sized bits
- 1 carrot, shredded
- 1 yellow zucchini, diced
- 4 fresh figs
- ¼ cup ground flaxseed
- 1 cup mixed green leaves
- 1 teaspoon sea salt

Directions:

1. Add kale to a bowl with avocado, lemon juice and sea salt. Massage together until kale wilts. Add in zucchini, carrot and 2 cups mixed green leaves. Fold in figs and remaining ingredients. Toss and serve.

Nutrition:

Calories 255

Fat 12.5 g

Carbs 35 g

Protein 6 g

Cucumber Avocado Toast

Preparation time: 15 minutes

Cooking time: 0 minutes

Servings: 2

Ingredients:

- 1 cucumber, sliced

- 2 sprouted (Essene) bread slices, toasted

- ¼ handful basil leaves, chopped

- 4 tablespoons avocado, mashed

- Salt and pepper, to taste

- 1 teaspoon lemon juice

Directions:

1. Combine lemon juice together with the mashed avocado, and then spread the mixture on two bread slices.

2. Top with cucumber slices along with the finely chopped basil leaves. Generously sprinkle with salt and pepper and enjoy!

Nutrition:

Calories 232

Fat 14 g

Carbs 24 g

Protein 5 g

Kale and Cucumber Salad

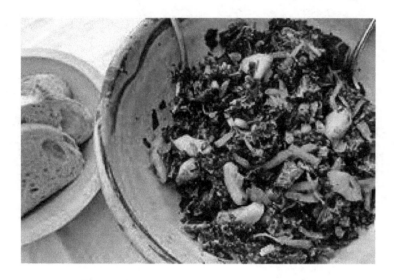

Preparation time: 15 minutes

Cooking time: 50 minutes

Servings: 2

Ingredients:

- 1 garlic clove

- 3 ½ oz fresh ginger

- 1/2 green Thai chili

- 1 ½ tablespoons sugar

- 1 ½ tablespoons fish sauce

- 1 ½ tablespoons vegetable oil

- 1 English cucumber, thinly sliced

- 1 bunch red Russian kale, ribs and stems removed; leaves torn into small pieces

- 1 Persian cucumber, thinly sliced

- 2 tablespoons fresh lime juice

- 1 small red onion, sliced

- 1 teaspoon sugar

- 2 tablespoons cilantro, chopped

- Salt, to taste

Directions:

1. Heat the broiler and broil ginger, with skin for 50 minutes, turning once. Let cool and slice. Blend chili, ginger, garlic, sugar, fish sauce, oil and 2 tablespoon water in a blender until paste forms.

2. Toss ¼ cup dressing and kale in a bowl and coat well. Massage with hands until kale softens.

3. Toss Persian and English cucumbers, lime juice, onion and sugar in a bowl and season with salt. Let it sit for 10 minutes.

4. Add the cucumber mixture to the bowl with kale and toss to combine. Top with cilantro and serve.

Nutrition:

Calories 160

Fat 8 g

Carbs 22 g

Protein 3 g

Mexican Quinoa

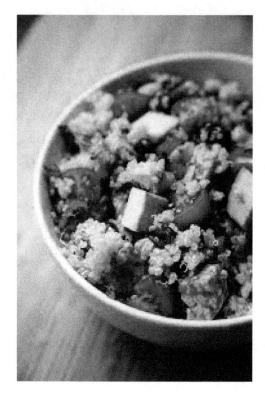

Preparation time: 15 minutes

Cooking time: 8 minutes

Servings: 4

Ingredients:

- 1 cup quinoa, uncooked and rinsed

- 1 ½ cup vegetable broth

- 3 cups diced tomatoes

- 2 cups frozen corn

- 1 cup fresh parsley, chopped

- 1 onion, chopped

- 3 cloves of garlic, minced

- 2 bell peppers, chopped

- 1 tablespoon paprika powder

- ½ tablespoon cumin

- 2 tablespoons olive oil

- 2 tablespoons lime juice

- 2 green onions, chopped

- salt and pepper

Directions:

1. Place a large pot over medium heat. Add olive oil. Cook onions for 3 minutes. Add garlic, bell peppers and cook for 5 minutes.

2. Add the remaining ingredients except for lime juice, green onions and parsley. Cover and cook for about 20 minutes, keep checking to make sure the quinoa doesn't stick and burn.

3. Add lime juice, green onions and parsley. Season the dish with salt and pepper before serving.

Nutrition:

Calories 231

Fat 17.8 g

Carbs 19 g

Protein 2 g

Mediterranean Parsley Salad

Preparation time: 15 minutes

Cooking time: 0 minutes

Servings: 2

Ingredients:

- ½ red onion, thinly sliced
- 1 cups parsley, chopped
- 1 Roma tomato, seeded and diced
- 6 mints, chopped
- 3 tablespoons currants, died
- 1 green chili, minced
- 1 tablespoon lemon
- 2 tablespoons olive oil
- 1/8 teaspoon sumac
- 1/8 teaspoon pepper, cracked
- ¼ teaspoon salt

Directions:

1. Mix lemon juice, olive oil, sumac, salt and pepper in a bowl and whisk to combine well. Toss parsley with the remaining ingredients in a separate bowl. Add the olive oil mixture to it and toss well and serve.

Nutrition:

Calories 110

Fat 8 g

Carbs 7 g

Protein 1 g

Tomatoes Parsley Salad

Preparation time: 15 minutes

Cooking time: 0 minutes

Servings: 2

Ingredients:

- 2 cups curly parsley leaves, packed
- 1 teaspoon garlic, minced
- 3/4 cup oil-packed sundried tomatoes, drained and julienned
- 2 tablespoons olive oil
- ½ cup basil leaves
- 2 tablespoons rice vinegar
- 1 shallot, minced
- 1 garlic clove, minced
- Salt and black pepper, to taste

Directions:

1. Wash parsley, dry and add to a bowl. Add garlic and tomatoes. Toss well. Wash basil and dry it. Add it to a blender and add vinegar, oil, salt and pepper to it. Blend until smooth.

2. Add garlic and shallots to the dressing. Add the dressing over salad and toss well. Divide among 6 salad plates and serve.

Nutrition:

Calories 245

Fat 19.8 g

Carbs 12 g

Protein 7 g

Lemon Parsley Quinoa Salad

Preparation time: 15 minutes

Cooking time: 0 minutes

Servings: 2

Ingredients:

- 1 tablespoon lemon juice
- 3 cups quinoa, cooked
- ¼ cup olive oil
- 1 ½ teaspoons lemon zest
- 1 cup Italian flat-leaf parsley, tightly packed
- ½ bell pepper, diced
- Salt and black pepper, to taste

Directions:

1. Cook quinoa according to package instructions. Put a splash of water and heat in a microwave. Mix lemon juice and lemon zest in a bowl and whisk in olive oil.

2. Add salt and pepper. Add parsley, rice and diced pepper. Mix well and season with salt and pepper. Enjoy!

Nutrition:

Calories 207

Fat 9 g

Carbs 28 g

Protein 2.6 g

Quinoa and Parsley Salad

Preparation time: 15 minutes

Cooking time: 0 minutes

Servings: 2

Ingredients:

- ½ cup quinoa, uncooked
- 1 cup water
- ¾ cup parsley leaves
- ½ cup celery, sliced
- ½ cup green onions, sliced
- 3 tablespoons fresh lemon juice
- ½ cup dried apricots, chopped
- 1 tablespoon agave syrup
- 1 tablespoon olive oil
- ¼ cup unsalted pumpkinseed kernels, toasted
- ¼ teaspoon salt
- ¼ teaspoon black pepper

Directions:

1. Add quinoa and water to a pan and bring to boil. Cover, reduce heat and simmer for 20 minutes. Add to a bowl and fluff with a fork. Add celery, parsley, onions and apricots.

2. Whisk olive oil, lemon juice, syrup, salt and black pepper. Add to quinoa mixture and toss well. Top with seeds and serve.

Nutrition:

Calories 238

Fat 8.6 g

Carbs 35 g

Protein 6 g

Broccoli and Mushroom Stir-Fry

Preparation time: 15 minutes

Cooking time: 20 minutes

Servings: 4

Ingredients:

- 2 cups broccoli, cut into small florets
- ¼cup red onion, chopped small
- 3 cloves garlic, minced
- 2 cups mushrooms, sliced
- ¼teaspoon crushed red pepper
- 2 teaspoons fresh ginger, grated
- 1 tablespoon olive oil
- ¼ cup water or broth
- ½ cup carrot, shredded
- ¼ cup cashews
- 2 tablespoons of rice wine vinegar
- 2 tablespoons soy sauce
- 1 tablespoon coconut sugar
- 1 tablespoon sesame seeds

Directions:

1. Pop a large skillet over medium heat and add the olive oil. Add the broccoli, onion, garlic, mushrooms, red pepper, ginger, and water.
2. Cook until the veggies are soft. Add the carrots, cashews, vinegar, soy, and coconut sugar. Stir well and cook for 2 minutes. Sprinkle with sesame seeds, then serve and enjoy.

Nutrition:

Calories: 133

Carbs: 9g

Fat: 8g

Lentil Vegetable Loaf

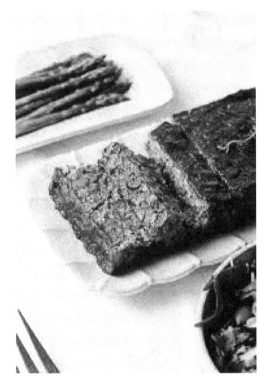

Preparation time: 15 minutes

Cooking time: 55 minutes

Servings: 4

Ingredients:

- 2 cups cooked lentils, drained well

- 1 tablespoon olive oil

- 1 small onion, diced

- 1 carrot, finely diced

- 1 stalk celery, diced

- 1 x 8 oz. package white or button mushrooms, cleaned and diced

- 3 tablespoons tomato paste

- 2 tablespoons soy sauce

- 1 tablespoon balsamic vinegar

- 1 cup old-fashioned oats, uncooked

- ½ cup almond meal

- 1 ½ teaspoons dried oregano

- 1/3 cup ketchup

- 1 teaspoon balsamic vinegar

- 1 teaspoon Dijon mustard

Directions:

1. Warm your oven to 400°F and grease a 5" x 7" loaf tin, then pops to one side. Add olive oil to a skillet and pop over medium heat.

2. Add the onion and cook for five minutes until soft. Add the carrots, celery, and mushrooms and cook until soft.

3. Grab your food processor and add the lentils, tomato paste, soy sauce, vinegar, oats, almond, and oregano. Whizz well until combined, then transfer to a medium bowl.

4. Pop the veggies into the food processor and pulse until combined. Transfer to the bowl. Stir everything together.

5. Move the mixture into the loaf pan, press down, and pop into the oven. Cook for 35 minutes, add the topping, then bake again for 15 minutes. Remove from the oven and allow about10 minutes to cool.

Nutrition:

Calories: 226

Carbs: 25g

Fat: 6g

Protein: 12g

Maple Glazed Tempeh with Quinoa and Kale

Preparation time: 15 minutes

Cooking time: 30 minutes

Servings: 5

Ingredients:

- 1 cup quinoa

- 1 ½ cups vegetable stock

- 8 oz. tempeh, cubed

- 2 tablespoons pure maple syrup

- 3 tablespoons dried cranberries

- 1 tablespoon fresh chopped thyme

- 1 tablespoon fresh chopped rosemary

- 1 tablespoon olive oil

- Juice of 1 orange

- 1 clove garlic, minced

- 4 oz. baby kale, chopped

Directions:

1. Preheat the oven to 400°F and use parchment to line on a paper baking sheet. Add the stock to a saucepan and pop over medium heat. Bring to the boil and add the quinoa.

2. Lower the heat, cover, and allow 15 minutes to simmer until cooked. Take a medium bowl, add the tempeh and pour the maple syrup and stir well until combined.

3. Place the tempeh onto the baking sheet and pop it into the oven for 15 minutes until brown. Meanwhile, grab a large bowl and add the rest of the ingredients. Stir well to combine.

4. Add the quinoa and cooked tempeh, season well with salt and pepper. Serve and enjoy.

Nutrition:

Calories: 321

Carbs: 35g

Fat: 12g

Protein: 16g

Slow Cooker Chili

Preparation time: 15 minutes

Cooking time: 9 hours

Servings: 12

Ingredients:

- 3 cups dry pinto beans
- 1 large onion, chopped
- 3 bell peppers, chopped
- 8 large green jalapeño peppers, dice after removing seeds by scraping out
- 2 x 14.5 oz. cans of diced tomatoes, or equivalent
- 1 tablespoon chili powder
- 2 tablespoons oregano flakes
- 1 tablespoon cumin powder
- 1 tablespoon garlic powder
- 3 bay leaves, freshly ground
- 1 teaspoon ground black pepper
- 1 tablespoon sea salt (or to taste)

Directions:

1. Put the beans into your large pan, filled with water, and leave to soak overnight. The next morning, drain and transfer to a 6-quart slow cooker.

2. Cover with salt and two inches of water. Cook on high for 6 hours until soft. Drain the beans and add the other ingredients. Stir well to combine. Cover and cook again within 3 hours on high. Serve and enjoy.

Nutrition:

Calories: 216

Carbs: 30g

Fat: 1g

Protein: 12g

Spicy Hummus Quesadillas

Preparation time: 5 minutes

Cooking time: 15 minutes

Servings: 4

Ingredients:

- 4 x 8" whole grain tortilla

- 1 cup hummus

- Your choice of fillings: spinach, sundried tomatoes, olives, etc.

- Extra-virgin olive oil for brushing

To serve:

- Extra hummus

- Hot sauce

- Pesto

Directions:

1. Put your tortillas on a flat surface and cover each with hummus. Add the fillings, then fold over to form a half-moon shape.

2. Pop a skillet over medium heat and add a drop of oil. Add the quesadillas and flip when browned. Repeat with the remaining quesadillas, then serve and enjoy.

Nutrition:

Calories: 256

Carbs: 25g

Fat: 12

Quinoa Lentil Burger

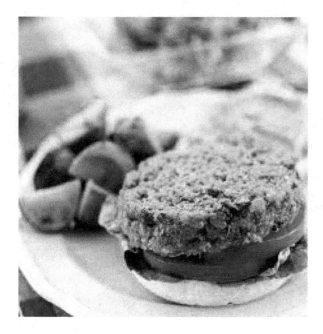

Preparation time: 5 minutes

Cooking time: 25 minutes

Servings: 4

Ingredients:

- 1 tablespoon + 2 teaspoons of olive oil

- ¼ cup red onion, diced

- 1 cup quinoa, cooked

- 1 cup cooked drained brown lentils

- 1 x 4 oz. green chilies, diced

- 1/3 cup oats, rolled

- ¼ cup flour

- 2 teaspoons corn starch

- ¼ cup panko breadcrumbs, whole-wheat

- ¼ teaspoon garlic powder

- ½ teaspoon cumin

- Paprika,1 teaspoon

- Salt and pepper

- 2 tablespoons Dijon mustard

- 3 teaspoons honey

Directions:

1. Put 2 teaspoons olive oil into your skillet over medium heat. Add the onion and cook for five minutes until soft. Grab a small bowl and add the honey and Dijon mustard.

2. Grab a large bowl and add the burger ingredients; stir well. Form into 4 patties with your hands. Put a tablespoon of oil into your skillet over medium heat.

3. Add the patties and cook for 10 minutes on each side. Serve with the honey mustard and enjoy!

Nutrition:

Calories: 268

Carbs: 33g

Fat: 8g

Protein: 10g

Spanish Vegetable Paella

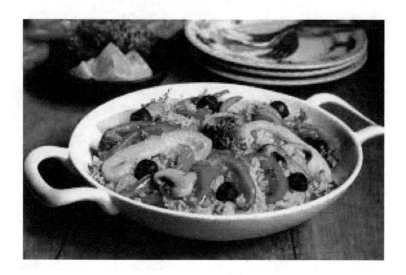

Preparation time: 15 minutes

Cooking time: 1 hour & 30 minutes

Servings: 6

Ingredients:

- 3 tablespoons virgin olive oil, divided

- 1 medium chopped fine yellow onion

- 1 ½ teaspoon fine sea salt, divided

- 6 garlic cloves, minced or pressed

- 2 teaspoons smoked paprika

- 15 oz. can dice tomatoes, drained

- 2 cups short-grain brown rice

- 15 oz. can garbanzo beans, rinsed & drained

- 3 cups vegetable broth

- 1/3 cup dry white wine/vegetable broth

- ½ teaspoon saffron threads, crumbled (optional)

- 14 oz. can quarter artichokes

- 2 red bell peppers, sliced into long, ½"-wide strips

- ½ cup Kalamata olives pitted and halved

- ¼ tsp ground black pepper

- ¼ cup chopped fresh parsley, + about 1 tablespoon more for garnish

- 2 tablespoons lemon juice

- Lemon wedges for garnish

- ½ cup frozen peas

Directions:

1. Preheat the oven to 350°F. Put 2 tablespoons of oil into your skillet and pop over medium heat. Add the onion and cook for five minutes until soft.

2. Add salt, garlic, and paprika—Cook for 30 seconds. Add the tomatoes, stir through and cook for 2 minutes. Add the rice, stir through, and cook again for a minute.

3. Add the garbanzo beans, broth, wine or stock, saffron, and salt, and bring to a boil. Cover and pop into the oven within 40 minutes until the rice has been absorbed. Line a baking sheet with parchment paper.

4. Grab a large bowl and add the artichoke, peppers, olives, 1 tablespoon olive oil, ½ Teaspoon of salt, and black pepper to taste. Toss to combine, then spread over the prepared baking sheet.

5. Pop into the oven and cook within 30 minutes. Remove from the oven and leave to cool slightly. Add the parsley, lemon juice, and seasoning as required. Toss.

6. Pop the rice onto a stove, turn up the heat and bake the rice for five minutes. Garnish and serve with the veggies.

Nutrition:

Calories: 437

Carbs: 60g

Fat: 16g

Protein: 10g

Tex-Mex Tofu & Beans

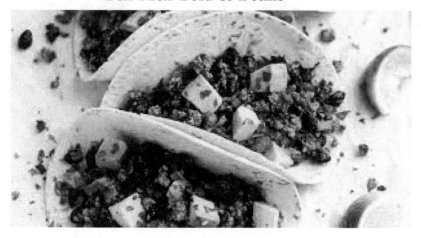

Preparation time: 25 minutes

Cooking time: 12 minutes

Servings: 2

Ingredients:

- 1 cup dry black beans

- 1 cup dry brown rice

- 1 14-oz. package firm tofu, drained

- 2 tbsp. olive oil

- 1 small purple onion, diced

- 1 medium avocado, pitted, peeled

- 1 garlic clove, minced

- 1 tbsp. lime juice

- 2 tsp. cumin

- 2 tsp. paprika

- 1 tsp. chili powder

- Salt and pepper to taste

Directions:

1. Cut the tofu into ½-inch cubes. Heat the olive oil in a skillet. Put the diced onions and cook until soft, for about 5 minutes.

2. Add the tofu and cook an additional 2 minutes, flipping the cubes frequently. Meanwhile, cut the avocado into thin slices and set aside.

3. Lower the heat and add in the garlic, cumin, and cooked black beans. Stir until everything is incorporated thoroughly, and then cook for an additional 5 minutes.

4. Add the remaining spices and lime juice to the mixture in the skillet. Mix thoroughly and remove the skillet from the heat.

5. Serve the Tex-Mex tofu and beans with a scoop of rice and garnish with the fresh avocado. Enjoy immediately, or store the rice, avocado, and tofu mixture separately.

Nutrition:

Calories: 315

Carbs: 27.8 g

Fat: 17 g

Protein: 12.7 g.

Spaghetti Squash Burrito Bowl

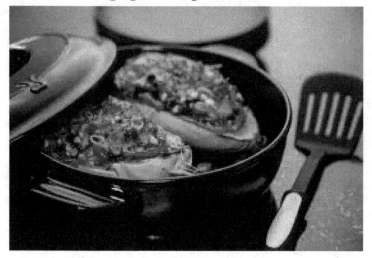

Preparation time: 5 minutes

Cooking time: 60 minutes

Servings: 4

Ingredients:

- 2 x 2 lb. spaghetti squash, halved and seeds removed

- 2 tablespoons olive oil

- Salt

- ground black pepper, to taste

- For the cabbage and black bean slaw:

- 2 cups purple cabbage, sliced thinly

- 15 oz. can black beans

- 2 tablespoons fresh lime juice

- 1 red bell pepper, sliced

- 1/3 cup chopped green onions

- 1/3 cup chopped fresh cilantro

- 1 teaspoon olive oil

- ¼ teaspoon salt

For the avocado salsa Verde:

- ¾ cup mild salsa Verde

- 1/3 cup fresh cilantro

- 1 avocado, diced

- 1 tbsp. fresh lime juice

- 1 chopped garlic clove

To garnish:

- Chopped fresh cilantro

- Crumbled feta

- Seasoned toasted pepitas

Directions:

1. Preheat your oven to 400°F and line a baking sheet with parchment paper. Place the spaghetti squash on top and drizzle with olive oil. Rub into the flesh

2. Sprinkle with salt and pepper and turn, so the cut sides are down. Roast for 40-60 minutes until soft.

3. Meanwhile, grab a medium bowl and add all the ingredients for the cabbage and black bean slaw. Stir well, then pop to one side.

4. Grab your blender, then add the salsa Verde ingredients. Whizz until smooth. Remove squash from the oven and use the fork to fluff up.

5. Divide between your serving bowls, then top with the slaw and the avocado salsa Verde. Top with the topping of your choice, then serve and enjoy.

Nutrition:

Calories: 301

Carbs: 21g

Fat: 17g

Protein: 8g

No-Egg Salad

Preparation time: 15 minutes

Cooking time: 0 minutes

Servings: 6

Ingredients:

- 1 (13-ounce) package firm tofu
- 1 celery stalk, finely chopped
- ¼ cup chives, finely chopped
- 1 tablespoon nutritional yeast
- 1 teaspoon turmeric
- ¼ teaspoon garlic powder
- ¼ teaspoon celery seed (optional)
- ½ teaspoon black salt (Kala namak)
- 2 tablespoon vegan mayonnaise
- 2 tablespoon dill pickle relish
- 1 tablespoon Dijon mustard
- 1 tablespoon fresh lemon juice
- Salt
- Freshly ground black pepper

Directions:

1. Crumble the tofu into a medium bowl with your hands. Then add the celery, chives, nutritional yeast, turmeric, garlic powder, celery seed (if using), and black salt and mix well.

2. In a small measuring cup or bowl, combine the vegan mayo, relish, mustard, and lemon juice to make a dressing. Put the dressing over the tofu batter and stir until everything is well combined.

3. Taste and season with salt and pepper, if desired. Enjoy.

Nutrition:

Calories: 87

Fat: 5g

Carbohydrate: 5g

Protein: 7g

Chickpea No Tuna Salad

Preparation time: 5 minutes

Cooking time: 0 minutes

Servings: 3

Ingredients:

- 1 (14-ounce) can chickpeas, drained and rinsed
- 2 celery stalks, finely chopped
- 2 scallions, coarsely chopped
- 2 tablespoons vegan mayonnaise
- Juice of ½ lemon
- 2 heaping teaspoons capers and brine
- 1 teaspoon dried dill or 1 handful fresh dill, chopped
- ½ teaspoon Dijon mustard
- ¼ teaspoon kelp flakes
- ¼ to ½ teaspoon salt
- Freshly ground black pepper

Directions:

1. In a medium bowl, combine the chickpeas, celery, scallions, mayo, lemon juice, capers, dill, mustard, kelp flakes, salt, and pepper.

2. Mix and mash everything together using a potato masher. Taste then flavors with additional salt, pepper, or lemon, if desired. Enjoy on its own, on top of a romaine or endive leaf, or with rice cakes.

Nutrition:

Calories: 193

Fat: 4g

Carbohydrate: 33g

Protein: 7g

Crunchy Rainbow Salad

Preparation time: 15 minutes

Cooking time: 0 minutes

Servings: 6

Ingredients:

- 4 cups shredded cabbage, red or green, or bagged slaw mix

- 2 cups cooked edamame

- 1 cup grated or shredded carrots

- ½ bunch cilantro, coarsely chopped

- 2 scallions, thinly sliced

- ½ cup dry roasted peanuts, chopped

- ¾ cup Sweet Peanut Dressing

- Salt

Directions:

1. Combine the cabbage, edamame, carrots, cilantro, scallions, and dry roasted peanuts in a medium bowl and mix well.

2. Add the peanut dressing and mix again, ensuring the dressing is evenly distributed—season with salt to taste.

Nutrition:

Calories: 276

Fat: 16g

Carbohydrate: 21g

Protein: 20g

Three-Bean Salad

Preparation time: 15 minutes

Cooking time: 0 minutes

Servings: 6

Ingredients:

- 1 (14-ounce) can kidney beans, drained & rinsed
- 1 (14-ounce) can chickpeas, drained and rinsed
- 1 (14-ounce) can white navy or cannellini beans, drained and rinsed
- ½ bunch parsley, coarsely chopped
- 2 celery stalks, finely chopped
- 1 red bell pepper, finely chopped
- 1 jalapeño pepper, minced (optional)
- 1 garlic clove, diced (optional)
- ¼ cup apple cider vinegar
- ¼ cup extra-virgin olive oil
- 1 tablespoon Dijon mustard
- 1 tablespoon maple syrup
- ½ teaspoon salt
- Freshly ground black pepper

Directions:

1. Combine the kidney beans, chickpeas, navy beans, parsley, celery, bell pepper, jalapeño pepper, and garlic (if used) in a medium bowl. Mix until evenly combined.

2. Put the apple cider vinegar, olive oil, mustard, maple syrup, and salt into the mixture and add as much black pepper as you'd like. Mix everything thoroughly, taste it, and adjust the seasoning with extra salt, if needed.

Nutrition:

Calories: 284

Fat: 10g

Carbohydrate: 40g

Protein: 11g

Greek Salad with Tofu Feta

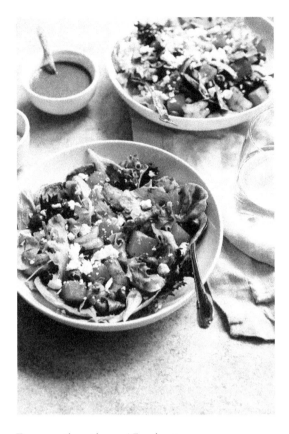

Preparation time: 15 minutes

Cooking time: 0 minutes

Servings: 6

Ingredients:

- 1 green bell pepper, coarsely chopped

- 1-pint cherry or grape tomatoes halved

- 1 small red onion, chopped

- 1 cucumber, chopped

- 1 (14-ounce) can butter beans, drained and rinsed

- ½ bunch parsley, coarsely chopped

- ½ cup pitted kalamata olives

- 1 garlic clove, minced

- Juice of 1 lemon

- 3 tablespoons red wine vinegar

- 3 tablespoons olive oil

- Tofu Feta

- 1 teaspoon salt

- Freshly ground black pepper

Directions:

1. In a medium bowl, combine the bell pepper, tomatoes, onion, cucumber, beans, parsley, olives, and garlic. Next, add the lemon juice, vinegar, and oil. Mix well.

2. Add the tofu feta (and any of the tofu marinade) to the salad. Season with salt and as much pepper as you would like, and then mix again.

Nutrition:

Calories: 142

Fat: 8g

Carbohydrate: 14g

Protein: 4g

Mushroom Lentil Soup

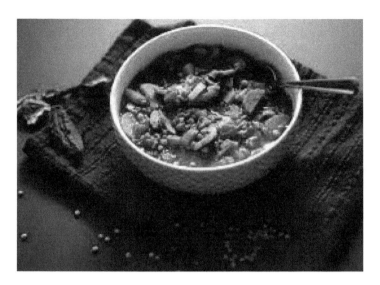

Preparation time: 15 minutes

Cooking time: 40 minutes

Servings: 6

Ingredients:

- 1 tablespoon olive oil
- 1 yellow onion, chopped
- 2 celery stalks, chopped
- 2 carrots, cut into thin rounds
- Pinch + ½ teaspoon salt, divided
- 3 garlic cloves, minced
- 2 cups cremini mushrooms, chopped
- 1 tablespoon dried rosemary
- 6 cups vegetable broth
- 1 cup brown lentils
- 4 cups chopped kale
- 3 tablespoons apple cider vinegar

- Freshly ground black pepper

Directions:

1. In a large stockpot, warm the oil over medium heat. Add the onion, celery, carrots, and a pinch of salt. Cook until the onions are slightly translucent, within 5 minutes.

2. Add the garlic and cook within 1 minute more; then add the mushrooms and rosemary. Stir everything together and cook for 5 minutes more or until the mushrooms have started to release liquid.

3. Add the vegetable broth and lentils. Boil; then reduce the heat to simmer. Cook within 30 minutes or until the lentils have softened. Stir in the kale and allow it to wilt for 1 or 2 minutes more.

4. Add the vinegar, remaining salt, and as much pepper as you'd like. Taste and adjust with additional salt or pepper, if desired.

Nutrition:

Calories: 205

Fat: 4g

Carbohydrate: 27g

Protein: 14g

Spicy Peanut Bowl

Preparation time: 25 minutes

Cooking time: 0 minutes

Servings: 4

Ingredients:

- 1 (8-ounce) package black bean noodles, cooked
- 2 cups cooked edamame beans
- 1 cup red cabbage, thinly sliced
- 1 cup carrots, grated or shredded
- 1 cup red peppers, finely chopped
- 1 cup mung bean or soybean sprouts
- ¼ cup dry roasted peanuts, coarsely chopped
- ¼ cup cilantro, coarsely chopped
- 4 scallions, coarsely chopped
- Sweet Peanut Dressing
- Hot sauce or red chili flakes (optional)

Directions:

1. Divide the noodles evenly among 4 food storage containers. Top each container of noodles with ½ cup of edamame, ¼ cup of cabbage, ¼ cup of carrots, ¼ cup of peppers, ¼ cup of sprouts, and 1 tablespoon of peanuts.

2. Garnish each container with cilantro and scallions. Top it with 3 tablespoons of peanut dressing and hot sauce or chili flakes (if using). Cover the remaining containers with airtight lids and store them in the refrigerator.

Nutrition:

Calories: 417

Fat: 11g

Carbohydrate: 69g

Protein: 14g

Plant-Strong Power Bowl

Preparation time: 25 minutes

Cooking time: 0 minutes

Servings: 4

Ingredients:

- 2 cups white or brown rice, cooked

- 1 (14-ounce) can of black beans, drained and rinsed

- 1 (14-ounce) can chickpeas, drained and rinsed

- 4 cups spinach, chopped

- 1 cucumber, chopped

- Microgreens, for garnish

- Lemon Parsley Dressing

Directions:

1. Divide the rice evenly among 4 food storage containers, and then add to each container ¼ cup of black beans, ¼ cup of chickpeas, 1 cup of spinach, and ¼ of the chopped cucumber.

2. Garnish each container with a small handful of microgreens. Serve.

Nutrition:

Calories: 514

Fat: 22g

Carbohydrate: 70g

Protein: 14g

Burrito Bowl

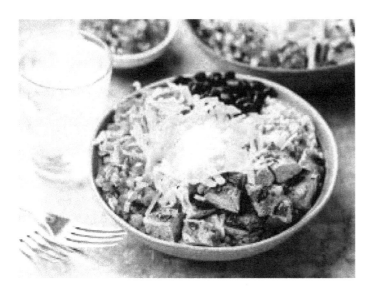

Preparation time: 15 minutes

Cooking time: 20 minutes

Servings: 4

Ingredients:

- 1 tablespoon olive oil

- 1 red onion, thinly sliced

- 1 bell pepper, thinly sliced

- Pinch salt

- 1 garlic clove, minced

- ½ teaspoon cumin

- 2 cups white or brown rice, cooked

- 1 (14-ounce) can pinto beans, drained & rinsed

- 4 cups spinach or arugula, chopped

- 1 avocado, chopped

- 4 scallions, coarsely chopped

- Hot sauce or salsa

- Cilantro Lime Dressing

Directions:

1. In a small skillet, warm the oil over medium-high heat. Add the onion, bell pepper, and a big pinch of salt. Sauté for 15 minutes or until the onions begin to caramelize slightly. Add the garlic and cumin and cook for 3 more minutes. Set aside.

2. Set out 4 food storage containers. To each container, add ½ cup of rice, ¼ of the bell pepper mixture, ¼ cup of beans, 1 cup of greens, and ¼ of the avocado.

3. Garnish each container with scallions and a hot sauce or salsa of your choice.

Nutrition:

Calories: 483

Fat: 31g

Carbohydrate: 50g

Protein: 10g

Harvest Bowl

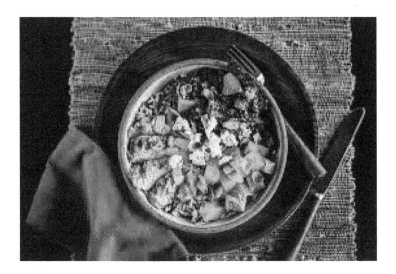

Preparation time: 15 minutes

Cooking time: 35 minutes

Servings: 4

Ingredients:

- 1 tablespoon olive oil

- 2 small sweet potatoes, chopped (about 2 cups)

- ½ teaspoon cinnamon

- ¼ teaspoon salt

- 2 cups wild rice, cooked

- 1 (14-ounce) can lentils, drained and rinsed

- 1 (14-ounce) can chickpeas, drained and rinsed

- 4 cups kale, thinly sliced and gently massaged

- 1 cup grated or shredded carrots

- ¼ cup hemp hearts

- ¼ cup raw sauerkraut (optional)

- Tahini Apple Cider Vinaigrette

Directions:

1. Warm oven to 400°F and lines a baking sheet with parchment paper. In a small bowl, mix the oil, potatoes, cinnamon, and salt.

2. Place the potatoes on the baking sheet and bake for 35 minutes or until the potatoes are nice and soft.

3. In each of 4 food storage containers, put ½ cup of rice, ¼ cup of lentils, ¼ cup of chickpeas, ¼ of the sweet potatoes, 1 cup of kale, and ¼ cup of carrots.

4. Garnish it with 1 tablespoon of hemp hearts and 1 tablespoon of sauerkraut (if using).

5. Finally, top it with 3 tablespoons of tahini vinaigrette. Cover the remaining containers with airtight lids and store them in the refrigerator.

Nutrition:

Calories: 563

Fat: 19g

Carbohydrate: 75g

Protein: 24g

Cauliflower Fried Rice

Preparation time: 15 minutes

Cooking time: 15 minutes

Servings: 6

Ingredients:

- 1 head cauliflower
- 1 tablespoon sesame oil
- 1 white onion, finely chopped
- 1 large carrot, finely chopped
- 4 garlic cloves, minced
- 2 cups frozen edamame or peas
- 3 scallions, sliced
- 3 tablespoons Bragg Liquid Aminos or tamari
- Salt
- Freshly ground black pepper

Directions:

1. Cut the cauliflower into florets and transfer them to a food processor. Process the cauliflower using the chopping blade and pulsing until the cauliflower is the consistency of rice. Set aside.

2. Warm a large skillet or wok over medium-high heat. Drizzle in the sesame oil and then add the onion and carrot, cooking until the carrots begin to soften about 5 minutes. Stir in the garlic and cook within another minute.

3. Add the cauliflower and edamame or peas. Heat until the cauliflower softens and the edamame or peas cook for about 5 minutes. Then add the scallions and liquid aminos or tamari. Mix well. Add in black pepper if desired.

Nutrition:

Calories: 117

Fat: 3g

Carbohydrate: 19g

Protein: 7g

Curried Quinoa Salad

Preparation time: 15 minutes

Cooking time: 15 minutes

Servings: 6

Ingredients:

- 1 tablespoon olive oil

- 1 garlic clove, minced

- 1 teaspoon-sized piece of ginger, minced

- 2 teaspoons curry powder

- 1 cup quinoa, rinsed under cold water using a fine-mesh strainer

- 1½ cups vegetable broth

- 1 (14-ounce) can chickpeas, drained and rinsed

- 2 celery stalks, finely chopped

- 1 cup carrots, shredded

- ¾ cup raisins

- 1 cup cilantro, chopped

- 3 tablespoons olive oil

- 3 tablespoons apple cider vinegar

- ½ teaspoon salt

- Freshly ground black pepper

Directions:

1. Warm-up oil over medium heat in a small saucepan. Add the garlic and ginger and cook for 1 minute. Add the curry powder and stir it.

2. Next, add the quinoa and toast it for about 5 minutes, stirring regularly. Then pour in the broth, turn the heat to high, and boil.

3. Adjust your heat to simmer, cover the saucepan, and cook for about 15 minutes or until the quinoa is light and fluffy.

4. Meanwhile, in a medium bowl, combine the chickpeas, celery, carrots, raisins, and cilantro. Once the quinoa is cooked, add it to the bowl as well. Then dress it with olive oil, vinegar, salt, and as much pepper as you'd like. Mix until well combined.

Nutrition:

Calories: 327

Fat: 12g

Carbohydrate: 50g

Protein: 8g

Lettuce Wraps with Smoked Tofu

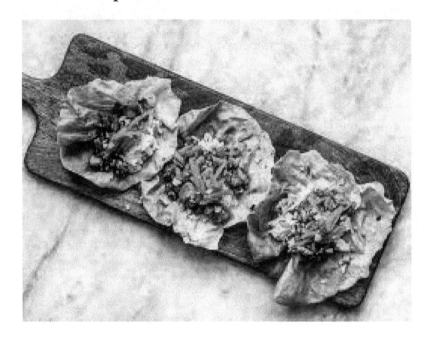

Preparation time: 15 minutes

Cooking time: 25 minutes

Servings: 4

Ingredients:

- 1 (13-ounce) package organic, extra-firm smoked tofu, drained and cubed

- 1 tablespoon coconut oil

- ½ cup yellow onion, finely chopped

- 3 celery stalks, finely chopped

- 1 red bell pepper, chopped

- Pinch salt

- 1 cup cremini mushrooms, finely chopped

- 1 garlic clove, minced

- ½ teaspoon ginger, minced

- 3 tablespoons Bragg Liquid Aminos, coconut aminos, or tamari

- ½ teaspoon red pepper flakes

- Freshly ground black pepper

- 8 to 10 large romaine leaves, washed and patted dry

Directions:

1. Preheat the oven to 350°F. Prepare a baking sheet lined using parchment paper or a silicone liner; then place the tofu cubes in a single layer. Bake the tofu cubes for 25 minutes, flipping them after 10 to 15 minutes. Set aside.

2. Meanwhile, warm the coconut oil in a nonstick sauté pan over medium-high heat. Add the onion, celery, bell pepper, and salt and cook for about 5 minutes or until the onions are slightly translucent.

3. Add the mushrooms, garlic, and ginger and sauté for about 5 minutes more or until the mushrooms begin to release water. Adjust the heat to medium, then put the aminos or tamari and the red pepper flakes.

4. Add the baked tofu cubes to the pan and sprinkle with pepper. Sauté for a few minutes more, until the tofu is coated with sauce and the veggies are tender.

5. To serve, scoop as much of the veggie and tofu mixture into each romaine leaf as you'd like.

Nutrition:

Calories: 160

Fat: 8g

Carbohydrate: 6g

Protein: 14g

Brussels Sprouts & Cranberries Salad

Preparation Time: 10minutes

Cooking Time: 0 minute

Servings: 6

Ingredients:

- 3 tablespoons lemon juice

- ¼ cup olive oil

- Salt and pepper to taste

- 1 lb. Brussels sprouts, sliced thinly

- ¼ cup dried cranberries, chopped

- ½ cup pecans, toasted and chopped

- ½ cup Parmesan cheese shaved

Direction

1. Mix the lemon juice, olive oil, salt, and pepper in a bowl. Toss the Brussels sprouts, cranberries, and pecans in this mixture. Sprinkle the Parmesan cheese on top.

Nutrition:

Calories 245

Fat 18.9 g

Carbohydrate 15.9 g

Protein 6.4 g

Quinoa Avocado Salad

Preparation Time: 15 minutes

Cooking Time: 4 minutes

Servings: 4

Ingredients:

- 2 tablespoons balsamic vinegar
- ¼ cup cream
- ¼ cup buttermilk
- 5 tablespoons freshly squeezed lemon juice, divided
- 1 clove garlic, grated
- 2 tablespoons shallot, minced
- Salt and pepper to taste
- 2 tablespoons avocado oil, divided
- 1 ¼ cups quinoa, cooked
- 2 heads endive, sliced
- 2 firm pears, sliced thinly
- 2 avocados, sliced
- ¼ cup fresh dill, chopped

Direction

1. Combine the vinegar, cream, milk, 1 tablespoon lemon juice, garlic, shallot, salt, and pepper in a bowl. Pour 1 tablespoon oil into a pan over medium heat. Heat the quinoa for 4 minutes.

2. Transfer quinoa to a plate. Toss the endive and pears in a mixture of remaining oil, remaining lemon juice, salt, and pepper. Transfer to a plate.

3. Toss the avocado in the reserved dressing. Add to the plate. Top with the dill and quinoa.

Nutrition:

Calories: 431

Fat: 28.5g

Carbohydrates: 42.7g

Chapter 4.   Dinner

Sweet Potato Bisque

Preparation time: 15minutes

Cooking time: 45minutes

Servings: 4

Ingredients:

- 2 sweet potatoes, peeled and sliced
- 2 cups frozen butternut squash
- 2 (14.5-ounce) cans full-fat coconut milk
- 1 medium yellow onion, sliced
- 1 teaspoon minced garlic (2 cloves)
- 1 tablespoon dried basil
- 1 tablespoon chili powder
- 1 tablespoon ground cumin
- 1/2 cup water
- Pinch salt
- Freshly ground black pepper

Directions:

1. Combine the sweet potatoes, butternut squash, coconut milk, onion, garlic, dried basil, chili powder, cumin, and water in a slow cooker; mix well.
2. Cook on low heat.
3. Blend the soup until it's nice and creamy.
4. Season with salt and pepper.

Nutrition:

Calories: 447

Total fat: 8g

Protein: 72g

Sodium: 346

Fat: 19g

Chickpea Medley

Preparation time: 5minutes

Cooking time: 15minutes

Servings: 4

Ingredients:

- 2 tablespoons tahini

- 2 tablespoons coconut amines

- 1 (15-ounce) can chickpeas or 1.1/2 cups cooked chickpeas, rinsed and drained

- 1 cup finely chopped lightly packed spinach

- Carrot, peeled and grated

Directions:

1. Merge together the tahini and coconut amines in a bowl.

2. Add the chickpeas, spinach, and carrot to the bowl. Stir well and serve at room temperature.

3. Simple Swap: Coconut amines are almost like a sweeter, mellower version of soy sauce. However, if you want to use regular soy sauce or tamari, just use 11/2 tablespoons and add a dash of maple syrup or agave nectar to balance out the saltiness.

Nutrition:

Calories: 437

Total fat: 8g

Protein: 92g

Sodium: 246

Fat: 19g

Pasta with Lemon and Artichokes

Preparation time: 10minutes

Cooking time: 20minutes

Servings: 4

Ingredients:

- 16 ounces linguine or angel hair pasta
- 1/4 cup extra-virgin olive oil
- 8 garlic cloves, finely minced or pressed
- 2 (15-ounce) jars water-packed artichoke hearts, drained and quartered
- 2 tablespoons freshly squeezed lemon juice
- 1/4 cup thinly sliced fresh basil
- 1 teaspoon sea salt
- Freshly ground black pepper

Directions:

1. Use a large pot of water to a boil over high heat and cook the pasta until al dente according to the directions on the package.

2. While the pasta is cooking, heat the oil in a skillet over medium heat and cook the garlic, stirring often, for 1 to 2 minutes until it just begins to brown. Toss the garlic with the artichokes in a large bowl.

3. When the pasta is done, drain it and add it to the artichoke mixture, then add the lemon juice, basil, salt, and pepper. Gently stir and serve.

Nutrition:

Calories: 237

Total fat: 7g

Protein: 52g

Sodium: 346

Fat: 19g

Roasted Pine Nut Orzo

Preparation time: 10minutes

Cooking time: 15minutes

Servings: 3

Ingredients:

- 16 ounces orzo
- 1 cup diced roasted red peppers
- 1/4 cup pitted, chopped Klamath olives
- 4 garlic cloves, minced or pressed
- 3 tablespoons olive oil
- 1.1/2 tablespoons squeezed lemon juice
- 2 teaspoons balsamic vinegar
- 1 teaspoon sea salt
- 1/4 cup pine nuts
- 1/4 cup packed thinly sliced or torn fresh basil

Directions:

1. Use a large pot of water to a boil over medium-high heat and add the orzo. Cook, stirring often, for 10 minutes, or until the orzo has a chewy and firm texture. Drain well.

2. While the orzo is cooking, in a large bowl, combine the peppers, olives, garlic, olive oil, lemon juice, vinegar, and salt. Stir well.

3. In a dry skillet toasts the pine nuts over medium-low heat until aromatic and lightly browned, shaking the pan often so that they cook evenly

4. Upon reaching the desired texture and add it to the sauce mixture within a minute or so, to avoid clumping.

Nutrition:

Calories: 537

Total fat: 7g

Protein: 72g

Sodium: 246

Fat: 19g

Banana and Almond Butter Oats

Preparation Time: 10 minutes

Cooking time: 5 minutes

Servings: 2

Ingredients:

- 1 cup gluten-free moved oats
- 1 cup almond milk
- 1 cup of water
- 1 teaspoon cinnamon
- 2 tablespoons almond spread
- 1 banana, cut

Directions:

1. Mix the water and almond milk to a bubble in a little pot. Add the oats and diminish to a stew.

2. Cook until oats have consumed all fluid. Blend in cinnamon. Top with almond spread and banana and serve.

Nutrition:

Calories: 112;

Fat: 10g;

Protein: 9g;

Carbohydrates: 54g;

Fiber: 15g;

Sugar: 5g;

Sodium: 180mg

Red Tofu Curry

Preparation time: 15 minutes

Cooking time: 65 minutes

Servings: 4

Ingredients:

- 1 1/2 tablespoon canola oil
- 1 package extra-firm tofu
- 3 cups baby carrots
- 2 cups peeled red
- 2 onions,
- 3 teaspoons garlic
- 1 piece ginger
- 1.1/2 cups water
- 1 cup canned unsweetened coconut milk
- 1.1/2 tablespoons red curry paste
- 1 vegetable bouillon cube
- 1/2 teaspoon salt
- Cooked rice, for serving
- Fresh cilantro, for garnish

Directions:

1. Heat the oil in a skillet. Place the tofu and brown.
2. Merge all the ingredients and mix well.
3. Cook on low heat
4. Present over rice and garnished with cilantro.

Nutrition:

Calories: 617

Total fat: 2g

Protein: 32g

Sodium: 563mg

Spicy Tomato-Lentil Stew

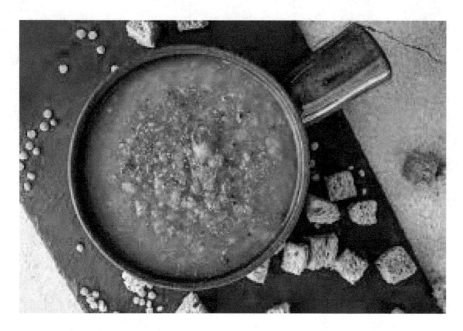

Preparation time: 15 minutes

Cooking time: 60 minutes

Servings: 5

Ingredients:

- 2 cups dry brown
- 1 can crushed tomatoes
- 1 can diced tomatoes
- 2 cups peeled potatoes
- 1 yellow onion
- 1/2 cup carrot
- 1/2 cup celery
- 2 tablespoons hot sauce
- 2 teaspoons garlic
- 2 teaspoons cumin
- 1 teaspoon chili

- 1/2 teaspoon coriander

- 1/4 teaspoon paprika

- 1 1/4 bay leaf

- pepper

- 4 bouillon cubes

Directions:

1. Merge all the ingredients and mix well.
2. Cook on low heat
3. Ready to serve.

Nutrition:

Calories: 517

Total fat: 2g

Protein: 32g

Sodium: 1,063mg

Fiber: 38g

Mixed-Bean Chili

Preparation time: 10minutes

Cooking time: 60 minutes

Servings: 4

Ingredients:

- 5 (15-ounce) cans your choice beans, drained and rinsed
- 1 (15-ounce) can diced tomatoes, with juice
- 1 (6-ounce) can tomato paste
- 1 cup water
- 1 green bell pepper, diced
- 2 cups stemmed and chopped kale
- 1/2 medium yellow onion, diced
- 2 tablespoons ground cumin
- 1 tablespoon chili powder
- 1 teaspoon minced garlic (2 cloves)
- 1 teaspoon cayenne pepper
- Pinch salt

Directions:

1. Place the beans, diced tomatoes, tomato paste, water, bell pepper, kale, onion, cumin, chili powder, garlic, and cayenne pepper in a slow cooker.
2. Season with salt and serve.

Nutrition:

Calories: 417

Total fat: 2g

Protein: 72g

Sodium: 463mg

Fiber: 10g

Butternut Squash Soup

Preparation time: 10minutes

Cooking time: 70 minutes

Servings: 4

Ingredients:

- 2 (10-ounce) packages frozen butternut squash
- 6 cups water
- 1 medium yellow onion, chopped
- 1 teaspoon minced garlic (2 cloves)
- 5 vegetable bouillon cubes
- 2 bay leaves
- 1/4 teaspoon freshly ground black pepper
- 1/8 teaspoon cayenne pepper
- 1 (8-ounce) package vegan cream cheese, cut into chunks

Directions:

1. Combine the butternut squash, water, onion, garlic, bouillon cubes, bay leaves, black pepper, and cayenne pepper in a slow cooker. Stir to mix.
2. Cook on low heat.
3. Remove the bay leaves.
4. Purée half of the soup using a blender.
5. Stir in the cream cheese. Cover and cook on low for 30 minutes longer.

Nutrition:

Calories: 617

Total fat: 2g

Protein: 82g

Sodium: 563mg

Fiber: 10g

Split-Pea Soup

Preparation time: 10minutes

Cooking time: 65 minutes

Servings: 5

Ingredients:

- 1-pound dried green split peas, rinsed
- 6 cups water
- 3 carrots, diced
- 3 celery stalks, diced
- 1 medium russet potato, peeled and diced
- 1 small yellow onion, diced
- 1.1/2 teaspoons minced garlic (3 cloves)
- 5 vegetable bouillon cubes
- 1 bay leaf
- Freshly ground black pepper

Directions:

1. Combine the split peas, water, carrots, celery, potato, onion, garlic, bouillon cubes, and bay leaf in a slow cooker; mix well.
2. Cook on low heat, and season with pepper.

Nutrition:

Calories: 817

Total fat: 2g

Protein: 82g

ng

Tomato Bisque

Preparation time: 10minutes

Cooking time: 65 minutes

Servings: 4

Ingredients:

- 2 (28-ounce) cans crushed tomatoes
- 1 (28-ounce) can whole peeled tomatoes, with juice
- 1 (15-ounce) can white beans, drained and rinsed
- 1/2 cup cashew pieces
- 2 vegetable bouillon cubes
- 1 tablespoon dried basil
- 2 teaspoons minced garlic (4 cloves)
- 3 cups water
- Pinch salt
- Freshly ground black pepper

Directions:

1. Combine the crushed tomatoes, whole peeled tomatoes, white beans, cashew pieces, bouillon cubes, dried basil, garlic, and water in a slow cooker.
2. Cook on low heat.
3. Blend the soup until smooth. Season with salt and pepper.

Nutrition:

Calories: 817

Total fat: 2g

Protein: 82g

Sodium:

Cheesy Potato-Broccoli Soup

Preparation time: 15minutes

Cooking time: 70minutes

Servings: 4

Ingredients:

- 2 pounds red or Yukon potatoes, chopped
- 1 (10-ounce) bag frozen broccoli
- 2 cups unsweetened nondairy milk
- 1 small yellow onion, chopped
- 1.1/2 teaspoons minced garlic (3 cloves)
- 3 vegetable bouillon cubes
- 4 cups water
- 1 cup melts able vegan Cheddar-cheese shreds (such as Diana or Follow Your Heart)
- Pinch salt
- Freshly ground black pepper

Directions:

1. Combine the potatoes, broccoli, nondairy milk, onion, garlic, bouillon cubes, and water in a slow cooker; mix well.
2. Cook on low heat.
3. Forty-five minutes before serving, use an immersion blender (or a regular blender, working in batches) to blend the soup until it's nice and creamy.
4. Stir in the vegan cheese, cover, and cook for another 45 minutes.
5. Season with salt and pepper.

Nutrition:

Calories: 517

Total fat: 2g

Protein: 92g

Sodium:

Vegetable Stew

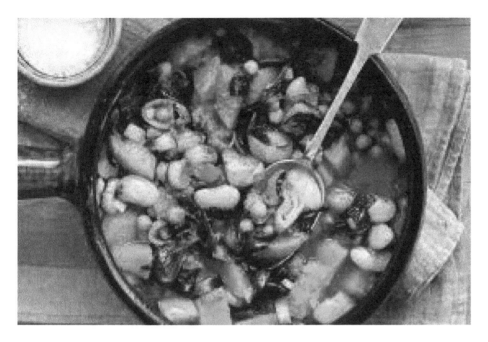

Preparation time: 15minutes

Cooking time: 65minutes

Servings: 4

Ingredients:

- 1 (28-ounce) can diced tomatoes, with juice
- 1 can white beans
- 1 cup diced green beans
- 2 medium potatoes, diced
- 1 cup frozen carrots and peas mix
- 1 small yellow onion, diced
- 1 (1-inch) piece ginger, peeled and minced
- 1 teaspoon minced garlic (2 cloves)
- 3 cups Vegetable Broth
- 2 teaspoons ground cumin
- 1/2 teaspoon red pepper flakes

- Juice of 1/2 lemon

- 1 cup dried pasta

- Pinch salt

- Freshly ground black pepper

- Pesto, for serving

Directions:

1. Combine the diced tomatoes, white beans, green beans, potatoes, carrots and peas mix, onion, ginger, garlic, vegetable broth, cumin, red pepper flakes, and lemon juice in a slow cooker.

2. Cook on low heat.

3. Pour with salt and pepper and serve with a dollop of pesto.

Nutrition:

Calories: 617

Total fat: 2g

Protein: 92g

Sodium: 356

Fat: 16g

Frijoles De La Olla

Preparation time: 15minutes

Cooking time: 65minutes

Servings: 4

Ingredients:

- 1-pound dry pinto beans, rinsed
- 1 small yellow onion, diced
- 1 jalapeño pepper, seeded and finely chopped
- 1.1/2 teaspoons minced garlic (3 cloves)
- 1 tablespoon ground cumin
- 1/2 teaspoon Mexican oregano (optional)
- 1 teaspoon red pepper flakes (optional)
- 4 cups water
- 2 tablespoons salt

Directions:

1. Place the beans, onion, jalapeño, garlic, cumin, oregano (if using), red pepper flakes (if using), water, and salt in a slow cooker.
2. Cook on low heat.

Nutrition

Total fat: 2g

Protein: 82g

Sodium: 346

Fat: 16g

Vegetable Hominy Soup

Preparation time: 15minutes

Cooking time: 30minutes

Servings: 4

Ingredients:

- 1 (28-ounce) can hominy, drained
- 1 (28-ounce) can diced tomatoes with green chills
- 5 medium red or Yukon potatoes, diced
- 1 large yellow onion, diced
- 2 cups chopped carrots
- 2 celery stalks, chopped
- 2 teaspoons minced garlic (4 cloves)
- 2 tablespoons chopped cilantro
- 1.1/2 tablespoons ground cumin
- 1.1/2 tablespoons seasoned salt
- 1 tablespoon chili powder
- 1 bay leaf
- 4 vegetable bouillon cubes
- 5 cups water
- Pinch salt
- Freshly ground black pepper

Directions:

1. Combine the hominy, diced tomatoes, potatoes, onion, carrots, celery, garlic, cilantro, cumin, seasoned salt, chili powder, bay leaf, vegetable bouillon, and water in a slow cooker; mix well. Cook on low heat.
2. . Remove the bay leaf. Season with salt and pepper.

Nutrition:

Calories: 417

Total fat: 2g

Protein: 72g

Sodium: 346

Lentil-Quinoa Chili

Preparation time: 15minutes

Cooking time: 30minutes

Servings: 4

Ingredients:

- 1/2 cup dry green lentils
- 1 can black beans
- 1/3 cup uncooked quinoa, rinsed
- 1 small yellow onion, diced
- 2 medium carrots, diced
- 2 teaspoons ground cumin
- 2 teaspoons chili powder
- 1.1/2 teaspoons minced garlic (3 cloves)
- 1 teaspoon dried oregano
- 3 vegetable bouillon cubes
- 1 bay leaf
- 4 cups water
- Pinch salt

Directions:

1. Place the lentils, black beans, quinoa, onion, carrots, cumin, chili powder, garlic, oregano, bouillon cubes, bay leaf, and water in a slow cooker; mix well.
2. Cook on low heat.
3. Remove the bay leaf, season with salt, and serve.

Nutrition:

Calories: 617

Total fat: 2g

Protein: 72g

Sodium: 346

Eggplant Curry

Preparation time: 15minutes

Cooking time: 35minutes

Servings: 5

Ingredients:

- 5 cups chopped eggplant
- 4 cups chopped zucchini
- 2 cups stemmed and chopped kale
- 1 (15-ounce) can full-fat coconut milk
- 1 (14.5-ounce) can diced tomatoes, drained
- 1 (6-ounce) can tomato paste
- 1 medium yellow onion, chopped
- 2 teaspoons minced garlic (4 cloves)
- 1 tablespoon curry powder
- 1 tablespoon gram masala
- 1/4 teaspoon cayenne pepper
- 1/4 teaspoon ground cumin
- 1 teaspoon salt
- Cooked rice, for serving

Directions:

1. Combine the eggplant, zucchini, kale, coconut milk, diced tomatoes, tomato paste, onion, garlic, curry powder, gram masala, cayenne pepper, cumin, and salt in a slow cooker; mix well.

2. Cook on low heat.

Nutrition:

Calories: 417

Total fat: 2g

Protein: 72g

Sodium: 346

Meaty Chili

Preparation time: 15minutes

Cooking time: 40minutes

Servings: 5

Ingredients:

- 1 tablespoon olive oil
- 2 packages of faux-ground-beef veggie crumble (such as Beyond Meat)
- 1 large red onion, chopped
- 1 large jalapeño pepper, seeded and chopped
- 2 1/2 teaspoons minced garlic
- 1 can diced tomatoes
- 1 can kidney beans
- 1 can black beans
- 1/2 cup frozen corn
- 1/4 cup chili powder
- 2 tablespoons ground cumin
- 1 teaspoon smoked paprika
- 1 vegetable bouillon cube
- 1.1/2 cups water

Directions:

1. Heat the olive oil in a sauté pan over medium-high heat. Add the veggie crumbles, onion, jalapeño, and garlic, and cook for 3 to 4 minutes, stirring occasionally.
2. Combine the veggie-crumble mixture, diced tomatoes, kidney beans, black beans, frozen corn, chili powder, cumin, smoked paprika, bouillon cube, and water in a slow cooker; mix well.
3. Cook on low heat.

Nutrition:

Calories: 547

Total fat: 8g

Protein: 62g

Sodium: 346

Black Bean Burgers

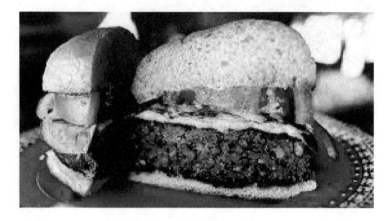

Preparation Time: 5 Minutes

Cooking Time: 20 Minutes

Servings: 4

Ingredients:

- 1 onion, diced

- 1/2 cup corn nibs

- 2 cloves garlic, minced

- 1/2 teaspoon oregano, dried

- 1/2 cup flour

- 1 jalapeno pepper, small

- 2 cups black beans, mashed & canned

- 1/4 cup breadcrumbs (vegan)

- 2 teaspoons parsley, minced

- 1/4 teaspoon cumin

- 1 tablespoon olive oil

- 2 teaspoons chili powder

- 1/2 red pepper, diced

- Sea salt to taste

Directions:

1. Set your flour on a plate, and then get out your garlic, onion, peppers and oregano, throwing it in a pan.

2. Cook over medium-high heat, and then cook until the onions are translucent.

3. Place the peppers in, and sauté until tender.

4. Cook for two minutes, and then set it to the side.

5. Use a potato masher to mash your black beans, and then stir in the vegetables, cumin, breadcrumbs, parsley, salt and chili powder, and then divide it into six patties.

6. Coat each side, and then cook until it's fried on each side.

Nutrition:

Calories: 211

Carbs: 12g

Fat: 7g

Protein: 12g

Dijon Maple Burgers

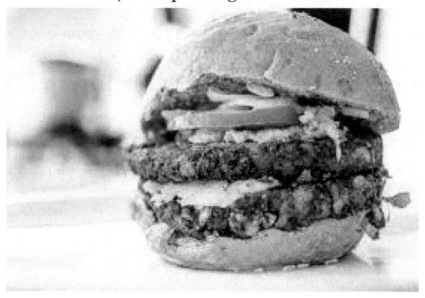

Preparation Time: 10 Minutes

Cooking Time: 40 Minutes

Servings: 12

Ingredients:

- 1 red bell pepper

- 19 ounces can chickpeas, rinsed & drained

- 1 cup almonds, ground

- 2 teaspoons Dijon mustard

- 1 teaspoon oregano

- 1/2 teaspoon sage

- 1 cup spinach, fresh

- 1 – 1/2 cups rolled oats

- 1 clove garlic, pressed

- 1/2 lemon, juiced

- 2 teaspoons maple syrup, pure

Directions:

1. Get out a baking sheet. Line it with parchment paper.

2. Cut your red pepper in half and then take the seeds out. Place it on your baking sheet, and roast in the oven while you prepare your other Ingredients:

3. Process your chickpeas, almonds, mustard and maple syrup together in a food processor.

4. Add in your lemon juice, oregano, sage, garlic and spinach, processing again. Make sure it's combined, but don't puree it.

5. Once your red bell pepper is softened, which should roughly take ten minutes, add this to the processor as well. Add in your oats, mixing well.

Nutrition:

Calories: 209

Carbs: 11g

Fat: 5g

Protein: 9g

Hearty Black Lentil Curry

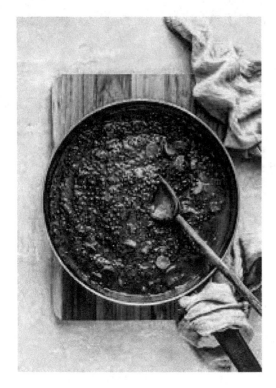

Preparation Time: 15 Minutes

Cooking Time: 6 Hours

Servings: 7

Ingredients:

- 1 cup of black lentils, rinsed and soaked overnight

- 14 ounces of chopped tomatoes

- 2 large white onions, peeled and sliced

- 1 1/2 teaspoon of minced garlic

- 1 teaspoon of grated ginger

- 1 red chili

- 1 teaspoon of salt

- 1/4 teaspoon of red chili powder

- 1 teaspoon of paprika

- 1 teaspoon of ground turmeric

- 2 teaspoons of ground cumin

- 2 teaspoons of ground coriander

- 1/2 cup of chopped coriander

- 4-ounce of vegetarian butter

- 1 fluid of ounce water

- 2 fluid of ounce vegetarian double cream

Directions:

1. Place a large pan over a moderate heat, add butter and let heat until melt.

2. Add the onion and garlic and ginger and let cook for 10 to 15 minutes or until onions are caramelized.

3. Then stir in salt, red chili powder, paprika, turmeric, cumin, ground coriander, and water.

4. Transfer this mixture to a 6-quarts slow cooker and add tomatoes and red chili.

5. Drain lentils, add to slow cooker and stir until just mix.

6. Plug in slow cooker; adjust cooking time to 6 hours and let cook on low heat setting.

7. When the lentils are done, stir in cream and adjust the seasoning.

8. Serve with boiled rice or whole wheat bread.

Nutrition:

Calories: 171

Carbs: 10g

Fat: 7g

Protein: 12g

Flavorful Refried Beans

Preparation Time: 15 Minutes

Cooking Time: 8 Hours

Servings: 8

Ingredients:

- 3 cups of pinto beans, rinsed
- 1 small jalapeno pepper, seeded and chopped
- 1 medium-sized white onion, peeled and sliced
- 2 tablespoons of minced garlic
- 5 teaspoons of salt
- 2 teaspoons of ground black pepper
- 1/4 teaspoon of ground cumin
- 9 cups of water

Directions:

1. Using a 6-quarts slow cooker, place all the Ingredients: and stir until it mixes properly.
2. Cover the top, plug in the slow cooker; adjust the cooking time to 6 hours, let it cook on high heat setting and add more water if the beans get too dry.
3. When the beans are done, drain them and reserve the liquid.
4. Mash the beans using a potato masher and pour in the reserved cooking liquid until it reaches your desired mixture.
5. Serve immediately.

Nutrition:

Calories: 198

Carbs: 22g

Fat: 7g

Protein: 19g

Smoky Red Beans and Rice

Preparation Time: 15 Minutes

Cooking Time: 5 Hours

Servings: 8

Ingredients:

- 30 ounces of cooked red beans
- 1 cup of brown rice, uncooked
- 1 cup of chopped green pepper
- 1 cup of chopped celery
- 1 cup of chopped white onion
- 1 1/2 teaspoon of minced garlic
- 1/2 teaspoon of salt
- 1/4 teaspoon of cayenne pepper
- 1 teaspoon of smoked paprika
- 2 teaspoons of dried thyme
- 1 bay leaf
- 2 1/3 cups of vegetable broth

Directions:

1. Using a 6-quarts slow cooker, all the Ingredients are except for the rice, salt, and cayenne pepper.
2. Stir until it mixes appropriately and then cover the top.
3. Plug in the slow cooker; adjust the cooking time to 4 hours, and steam on a low heat setting.
4. Then pour in and stir the rice, salt, cayenne pepper and continue cooking for an additional 2 hours at a high heat setting.

Nutrition:

Calories: 234

Carbs: 13g

Fat: 7g

Protein: 19g

Spicy Black-Eyed Peas

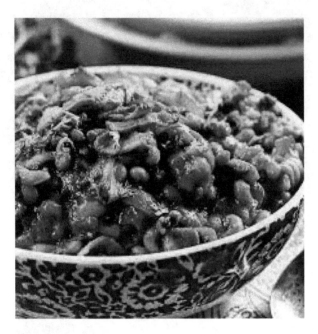

Preparation Time: 15 Minutes

Cooking Time: 60 Minutes

Servings: 8

Ingredients:

- 32-ounce black-eyed peas, uncooked
- 1 cup of chopped orange bell pepper
- 1 cup of chopped celery
- 8-ounce of chipotle peppers, chopped
- 1 cup of chopped carrot
- 1 cup of chopped white onion
- 1 teaspoon of minced garlic
- 3/4 teaspoon of salt
- 1/2 teaspoon of ground black pepper
- 2 teaspoons of liquid smoke flavoring

- 2 teaspoons of ground cumin

- 1 tablespoon of adobo sauce

- 2 tablespoons of olive oil

- 1 tablespoon of apple cider vinegar

- 4 cups of vegetable broth

Directions:

1. Place a medium-sized non-stick skillet pan over an average temperature of heat; add the bell peppers, carrot, onion, garlic, oil and vinegar.

2. Stir until it mixes properly and let it cook for 5 to 8 minutes or until it gets translucent.

3. Transfer this mixture to a 6-quarts slow cooker and add the peas, chipotle pepper, adobo sauce and the vegetable broth.

4. Stir until mixes properly and cover the top.

5. Plug in the slow cooker; adjust the cooking time to 8 hours and let it cook on the low heat setting or until peas are soft.

Nutrition:

Calories: 211

Carbs: 22g

Fat: 7g

Protein: 19g

Creamy Artichoke Soup

Preparation Time: 5 Minutes

Cooking Time: 40 Minutes

Servings: 4

Ingredients:

- 1 can artichoke hearts, drained
- 3 cups vegetable broth
- 2 tablespoon lemon juice
- 1 small onion, finely cut
- 2 cloves garlic, crushed
- 3 tablespoons olive oil
- 2 tablespoon flour
- 1/2 cup vegan cream

Directions:

1. Gently sauté the onion and garlic in some olive oil.
2. Add the flour, whisking constantly, and then add the hot vegetable broth slowly, while still whisking. Cook for about 5 minutes.
3. Blend the artichoke, lemon juice, salt and pepper until smooth. Add the puree to the broth mix, stir well, and then stir in the cream.
4. Cook until heated through. Garnish with a swirl of vegan cream or a sliver of artichoke.

Nutrition:

Calories: 211

Carbs: 12g

Fat: 7g

Protein: 11g

Super Rad-ish Avocado Salad

Preparation Time: 10 Minutes

Cooking Time: 25 Minutes

Servings: 2

Ingredients:

- 6 shredded carrots
- 6 ounces diced radishes
- 1 diced avocado
- 1/3 cup ponzu

Directions:

1. Bring all the above ingredients together in a serving bowl and toss.
2. Enjoy!

Nutrition:

Calories: 211

Carbs: 9g

Fat: 7g

Protein: 12g

Beauty School Ginger Cucumbers

Preparation Time: 10 Minutes

Cooking Time: 5 Minutes

Servings: 2

Ingredients:

- 1 sliced cucumber
- 3 teaspoon rice wine vinegar
- 1 1/2 tablespoon sugar
- 1 teaspoon minced ginger

Directions:

1. Bring all of the above ingredients together in a mixing bowl, and toss the ingredients well.
2. Enjoy!

Nutrition:

Calories: 210

Carbs: 14g

Fat: 7g

Protein: 19g

Mushroom Salad

Preparation Time: 10 Minutes

Cooking Time: 20 Minutes

Servings: 2

Ingredients:

- 1 tablespoon butter
- 1/2-pound cremini mushrooms, chopped
- 2 tablespoons extra-virgin olive oil
- Salt and black pepper to taste
- 2 bunches arugula
- 4 slices prosciutto
- 1 tablespoon apple cider vinegar
- 4 sundried tomatoes in oil, drained and chopped
- Fresh parsley leaves, chopped

Directions:

1. Heat a pan with butter and half of the oil.
2. Add the mushrooms, salt, and pepper. Stir-fry for 3 minutes. Reduce heat. Stir again, and cook for 3 minutes more.
3. Add rest of the oil and vinegar. Stir and cook for 1 minute.
4. Place arugula on a platter, add prosciutto on top, add the mushroom mixture, sundried tomatoes, more salt and pepper, parsley, and serve.

Nutrition:

Calories: 191

Carbs: 6g

Fat: 7g

Protein: 17g

Red Quinoa and Black Bean Soup

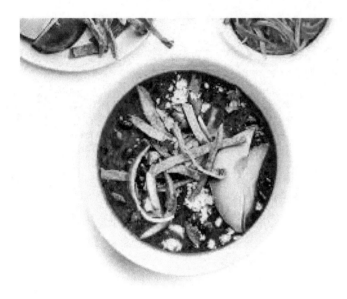

Preparation Time: 5 Minutes

Cooking Time: 40 Minutes

Servings: 6

Ingredients:

- 1/4 cup red quinoa

- 4 minced garlic cloves

- 1/2 tablespoon coconut oil

- 1 diced jalapeno

- 3 cups diced onion

- 2 teaspoon cumin

- 1 chopped sweet potato

- 1 teaspoon coriander

- 1 teaspoon chili powder

- 5 cups vegetable broth

- 15 ounces' black beans

- 1/2 teaspoon cayenne pepper

- 2 cups spinach

Directions:

1. Begin by bringing the quinoa into a saucepan to boil with two cups of water. Allow the quinoa to simmer for twenty minutes. Next, remove the quinoa from the heat.

2. To the side, heat the oil, the onion, and the garlic together in a large soup pot.

3. Add the jalapeno and the sweet potato and sauté for an additional seven minutes.

4. Next, add all the spices and the broth and bring the soup to a simmer for twenty-five minutes. The potatoes should be soft.

5. Before serving, add the quinoa, the black beans, and the spinach to the mix. Season, and serve warm. Enjoy.

Nutrition:

Calories: 211

Carbs: 22g

Fat: 7g

Protein: 19g

October Potato Soup

Preparation Time: 5 Minutes

Cooking Time: 20 Minutes

Servings: 3

Ingredients:

- 4 minced garlic cloves
- 2 teaspoon coconut oil
- 3 diced celery stalks
- 1 diced onion
- 2 teaspoon yellow mustard seeds
- 5 diced Yukon potatoes
- 6 cups vegetable broth
- 1 teaspoon oregano
- 1 teaspoon paprika
- 1/2 teaspoon cayenne pepper
- 1 teaspoon chili powder
- Salt and pepper to taste

Directions:

1. Begin by sautéing the garlic and the mustard seeds together in the oil in a large soup pot.
2. Next, add the onion and sauté the mixture for another five minutes.
3. Add the celery, the broth, the potatoes, and all the spices, and continue to stir.
4. Allow the soup to simmer for thirty minutes without a cover.
5. Next, Position about three cups of the soup in a blender, and puree the soup until you've reached a smooth consistency. Pour this back into the big soup pot, stir, and serve warm. Enjoy.

Nutrition:

Calories: 203

Carbs: 12g

Fat: 7g

Protein: 9g

Rice with Asparagus and Cauliflower

Preparation Time: 5 Minutes

Cooking Time: 20 Minutes

Servings: 2

Ingredients:

- 3 ounces' asparagus
- 3 ounces' cauliflower, chopped
- 2 ounces' tomato sauce
- 1/2 cup of brown rice
- 3/4 cup of water
- 1/3 teaspoon salt
- 1/4 teaspoon ground black pepper
- 1/4 teaspoon garlic powder
- 1 tablespoon olive oil

Directions:

1. Take a medium saucepan, place it over medium heat, add oil, add asparagus and cauliflower and then sauté for 5 to 7 minutes until golden brown.
2. Season with garlic powder, salt, and black pepper, stir in tomato sauce, and then cook for 1 minute.
3. Add rice, pour in water, stir until mixed, cover with a lid and cook for 10 to 12 minutes until rice has absorbed all the liquid and become tender.
4. When done, remove the pan from heat, fluff rice with a fork, and then serve.

Nutrition:

Calories: 257

Carbs: 4g

Fat: 4g

Protein: 40g

Spaghetti with Tomato Sauce

Preparation Time: 5 Minutes

Cooking Time: 15 Minutes

Servings: 2

Ingredients:

- 4 ounces' spaghetti
- 2 green onions, greens, and whites separated
- 1/8 teaspoon coconut sugar
- 3 ounces' tomato sauce
- 1 tablespoon olive oil
- 1/3 teaspoon salt
- 1/4 teaspoon ground black pepper

Directions:

1. Prepare the spaghetti, and for this, cook it according to the Directions on the packet and then set aside.
2. Then take a skillet pan, place it over medium heat, add oil and when hot, add white parts of green onions and cook for 2 minutes until tender.
3. Add tomato sauce, season with salt and black pepper and bring it to a boil.
4. Switch heat to medium-low level, simmer sauce for 1 minute, then add the cooked spaghetti and toss until mixed.
5. Divide spaghetti between two plates, and then serve.

Nutrition:

Calories: 265

Carbs: 8g

Fat: 2g

Protein: 7g

Crispy Cauliflower

Preparation Time: 5 Minutes

Cooking Time: 15 Minutes

Servings: 2

Ingredients:

- 6 ounces of cauliflower florets
- 1/2 of zucchini, sliced
- 1/2 teaspoon of sea salt
- 1/2 tablespoon curry powder
- 1/4 teaspoon maple syrup
- 2 tablespoons olive oil

Directions:

1. Switch on the oven, then set it to 450 degrees F and let it preheat.
2. Meanwhile, take a medium bowl, add cauliflower florets and zucchini slices, add remaining ingredients reserving 1 tablespoon oil, and toss until well coated.
3. Take a medium skillet pan, place it over medium-high heat, add remaining oil and wait until it gets hot.
4. Spread cauliflower and zucchini in a single layer and sauté for 5 minutes, tossing frequently.
5. Then transfer the pan into the oven and then bake for 8 to 10 minutes until vegetables have turned golden brown and thoroughly cooked, stirring halfway.

Nutrition:

Calories: 161

Carbs: 2g

Fat: 2g

Protein: 7g

Avocado Toast with Chickpeas

Preparation Time: 5 Minutes

Cooking Time: 5 Minutes

Servings: 2

Ingredients:

- 1/2 of avocado, peeled, pitted
- 4 tablespoons canned chickpeas, liquid reserved
- 1 tablespoon lime juice
- 1 teaspoon apple cider vinegar
- 2 slices of bread, toasted
- 1/4 teaspoon salt
- 1/4 teaspoon paprika
- 1 teaspoon olive oil

Directions:

1. Take a medium skillet pan, place it over medium heat, add oil and when hot, add chickpeas and cook for 2 minutes.
2. Sprinkle 1/8 teaspoon each salt and paprika over chickpeas, toss to coat, and then remove the pan from heat.
3. Place avocado in a bowl, mash by using a fork, drizzle with lime juice and vinegar and stir until well mixed.
4. Spread mashed avocado over bread slices, scatter chickpeas on top and then serve.

Nutrition:

Calories: 235

Carbs: 5g

Fat: 5g

Protein: 31g

Green Onion Soup

Preparation Time: 5 Minutes

Cooking Time: 12 Minutes

Servings: 2

Ingredients:

- 6 green onions, chopped
- 7 ounces diced potatoes
- 1/3 teaspoon salt
- 2 tablespoons olive oil
- 1/4 cup vegetable broth
- 1/4 teaspoon ground white pepper
- 1/4 teaspoon ground coriander

Directions:

1. Take a small pan, place potato in it, cover with water, and then place the pan over medium heat.
2. Boil the potato until cooked and tender, and when done, drain the potatoes and set aside until required.
3. Return saucepan over low heat, add oil and add green onions and cook for 5 minutes until cooked.
4. Season with salt, pepper, and coriander, add potatoes, pour in vegetable broth, stir until mixed and bring it to simmer.
5. Then remove the pan from heat and blend the mixture by using an immersion blender until creamy.
6. Taste to adjust seasoning, then ladle soup into bowls and then serve.

Nutrition:

Calories: 191

Carbs: 1g

Fat: 1g

Protein: 15g

Potato Soup

Preparation Time: 5 Minutes

Cooking Time: 12 Minutes

Servings: 2

Ingredients:

- 2 potatoes, peeled, cubed
- 1/3 teaspoon salt
- 1/2 cup vegetable broth
- 3/4 cup of water
- 1/8 teaspoon ground black pepper
- 1 tablespoon Cajun seasoning

Directions:

1. Take a small pan, place potato cubes in it, cover with water and vegetable broth, and then place the pan over medium heat.
2. Boil the potato until cooked and tender, and when done, remove the pan from heat and blend the mixture by using an immersion blender until creamy.
3. Return pan over medium-low heat, add remaining Ingredients: stir until mixed and bring it to a simmer.
4. Taste to adjust seasoning, then ladle soup into bowls and then serve.

Nutrition:

Calories: 203

5g

Teriyaki Eggplant

Preparation Time: 5 Minutes

Cooking Time: 15 Minutes

Servings: 2

Ingredients:

- 1/2-pound eggplant
- 1 green onion, chopped
- 1/2 teaspoon grated ginger
- 1/2 teaspoon minced garlic
- 1/3 cup soy sauce
- 1 tablespoon coconut sugar
- 1/2 tablespoon apple cider vinegar
- 1 tablespoon olive oil

Directions:

1. Prepare vegan teriyaki sauce and for this, take a medium bowl, add ginger, garlic, soy sauce, vinegar, and sugar in it and then whisk until sugar has dissolved completely.
2. Cut eggplant into cubes, add them into vegan teriyaki sauce, toss until well coated and marinate for 10 minutes.
3. When ready to cook, take a grill pan, place it over medium-high heat, grease it with oil, and when hot, add marinated eggplant.
4. Cook for 3 to 4 minutes per side until nicely browned and beginning to charred, drizzling with excess marinade frequently and transfer to a plate.
5. Sprinkle green onion on top of the eggplant and then serve.

Nutrition:

Calories: 132

Carbs: 4g

Fat: 4g

Protein: 13g

Broccoli Stir-Fry with Sesame Seeds

Preparation Time: 10 Minutes

Cooking Time: 8 Minutes

Servings: 4

Ingredients:

- Two tablespoons extra-virgin olive oil (optional)
- One tablespoon grated fresh ginger
- cups broccoli florets
- ¼teaspoon sea salt (optional)
- Two garlic cloves, minced
- Two tablespoons toasted sesame seeds

Directions:

1. Heat the olive oil (if desired) in a large nonstick skillet over medium-high heat until shimmering.
2. Fold in the ginger, broccoli, and sea salt (if desired) and stir-fry for 5 to 7 minutes, or until the broccoli is browned.
3. Cook the garlic until tender, about 30 seconds.
4. Sprinkle with the sesame seeds and serve warm.

Nutrition:

Calories: 135

Fat: 10.9g

Carbs: 9.7g

Protein: 4.1g

Fiber: 3.3g

Bream

Preparation time: 10minutes

Cooking time: 60minutes

Servings: 4

Ingredients:

- Olive oil cooking spray
- 2 medium zucchinis, cut into 1/2inch-thick rounds
- 2 gold potatoes, thinly sliced
- 4 tomatoes, sliced
- 1.3/4 cups tomato sauce
- 10 garlic cloves cut into large chunks
- 1.1/2 tablespoons olive oil
- 4 teaspoons dried basil
- 2 teaspoons dried oregano
- Teaspoon sea salt

Directions:

1. In a large bowl, combine the zucchini, potatoes, tomatoes, tomato sauce, garlic, olive oil, basil, oregano, and salt and stir well. Pour the vegetable into the dish.

2. Bake for 30 minutes, stir well, and bake for another 30 minutes, or until the potatoes are tender. Stir again and serve.

Nutrition:

Calories: 337

Total fat: 8

Protein: 82g

Sodium: 346

Fat: 19g

Green-Glory Soup (Pressure- Pot)

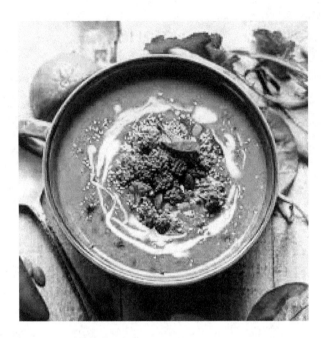

Preparation time: 10 minutes

Cooking time: 15 minutes

Servings: 4

Ingredients:

- 1 head cauliflower (florets)

- 1 onion (diced)

- 2 cloves garlic (minced)

- 1 cup spinach (fresh or frozen)

- 1 bay leaf (crumbled)

- 1 cup coconut milk

- 4 cups vegetable stock

- Salt and pepper to taste

- Herbs for garnish (optional)

- 1/2 cup coconut oil

Directions:

1. In a pressure pot on "sauté" mode, sauté onions and garlic until onions are browned. Once cooked, add the cauliflower and bay leaf and cook for about 5 minutes, stirring occasionally.

2. Add the spinach and continue cooking and stirring for 5 minutes.

3. Pour in the vegetable stock and set the timer for 10 minutes on high pressure to let the mix come to a boil; then allow quick pressure release and add the coconut milk.

4. Season with garnishes of choice as well as salt and pepper. Turn off the pot and mix the soup until it becomes thick and creamy with a hand blender.

Nutrition:

Calories: 114

Total fat: 9g

Saturated fat: 5g

Sodium: 128mg

Carbs: 19g

Fiber: 8g

Protein: 6g

Veggie Soup (Pressure- Pot)

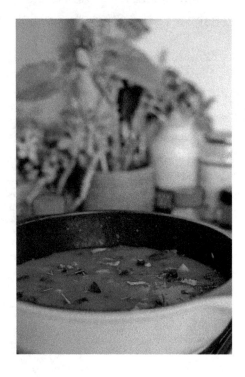

Preparation time: 5 minutes

Cooking time: 10 minutes

Servings: 4

Ingredients:

- 2 tbsp. olive oil

- 1 onion (medium, chopped)

- 3 tbsp. parsley (fresh, minced)

- 1 clove of garlic (minced)

- 3 (14.5 oz.) cans vegetable broth

- 4 cups tomatoes (chopped)

- 1 cup celery (chopped)

- 1 cup carrots (sliced)

- 1 zucchini (halved and sliced)

- 2 tsp. basil (dried, crushed)

- 1/2 tsp. salt

- 1/2 tsp. Italian seasoning

- 1 tsp. red pepper flakes (crushed)

- 5 cups kale leaves (chopped)

Directions:

1. Heat pot on "sauté" mode until it says "hot"; then adds the oil.

2. Attach the onion, and cook until it is tender. Add the parsley and garlic, stirring constantly for 30 seconds; then add the vegetable broth.

3. Stir in the celery, tomato, zucchini, carrots, Italian seasoning, and red pepper to the pot and turn off the heat. Close the lid.

4. Turn the steam option to "sealing," selecting high pressure for 6 minutes. When done, turn the cooker off again, choosing the quick pressure release option; then select "sauté."

5. Add kale, stirring for 3 minutes or so until the soup comes to a boil. Turn the cooker off and serve.

Nutrition:

Calories: 134

Total fat: 9g

Saturated fat: 5g

Sodium: 138mg

Carbs: 26g

Fiber: 8g

Protein: 6g

Creamy Italian Herb Soup

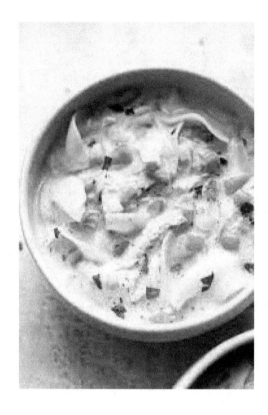

Preparation time: 10 minutes

Cooking time: 30 minutes

Servings: 4

Ingredients:

- 2 cans full fat coconut milk
- 1/2 cup coconut cream
- 1/4 cup fresh parsley
- 1 cup broccoli florets
- 1 cup veggie broth
- 1 tbsp. olive oil
- 1 tsp. nutritional yeast

- 1 finely chopped onion

- 2 cloves minced garlic

- 1 cup fresh Italian herbs (basil, oregano, rosemary, thyme, and sage)

- Salt and black pepper to taste

Directions:

1. Caramelize onion and garlic in a large cooking pan over medium heat.

2. Add Italian herbs, stir, and adding coconut milk while stirring.

3. Add remaining ingredients with salt and pepper to taste and cook for 30 minutes.

4. You can blend it after cooking or eat it when it's the right temperature.

5. If you want to store and freeze, you have to blend it.

6. Either transfers it directly to a heat safe blender, or let it cool, then blends until smooth.

Nutrition:

Calories: 124

Total fat: 9g

Saturated fat: 5g

Sodium: 118mg

Carbs: 16g

Fiber: 8g

Protein: 6g

Cauliflower Soup (Instant Pot)

Preparation time: 10 minutes

Cooking time: 30 minutes

Servings: 4

Ingredients:

- 3 cups vegetable stock
- 2 tsp. thyme powder
- 1/2 tsp. match green tea powder
- 1 head cauliflower (about 2.5 cups, florets)
- 1 tbsp. olive oil
- 5 garlic cloves (minced)
- Salt and pepper to taste

Directions:

1. In an instant pressure pot, add the vegetable stock, thyme, and match powder on medium heat. Bring to a boil.
2. Add the cauliflower and set timer for 10 minutes on high pressure, allowing for quick pressure release when finished.
3. In a saucepan, add garlic and olive oil until tender and you can smell it; then add it to the pot along with salt and cook for 1 to 2 minutes.
4. Turn off the heat and. blend the soup and creamy with a blender.

Nutrition:

Calories: 114

 Total fat: 9g

Saturated fat: 5g

Sodium: 128mg

Carbs: 18g

Fiber: 8g

Protein: 6g

Lasagna Soup

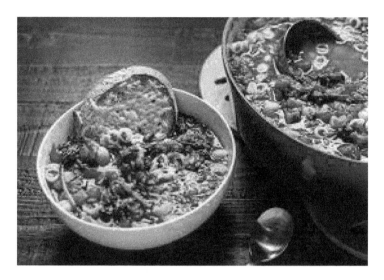

Preparation time: 5 minutes

Cooking time: 30 minutes

Servings: 5

Ingredients:

- Vegetable broth – 2 cups

- Portobello mushrooms, gills removed and finely diced – 8 ounces

- Onion powder – 1 teaspoon

- Crushed tomatoes – 28 ounces

- Diced tomatoes – 28 ounces

- Olive oil – 2 tablespoons

- Garlic, minced – 4 cloves

- Basil, fresh, chopped - .33 cup

- Nutritional yeast – 2 tablespoons

- Sea salt – 1 teaspoon

- Lentil Lasagna noodles (Explore Cuisine) – 8 ounces

- Vegan mozzarella shreds - .66 cup

- Thyme, dried – 1 teaspoon

Directions:

1. Pour the olive oil and allow it to heat over medium-high. Add in the diced mushrooms and cook while stirring regularly for eight minutes. Pour the diced tomatoes, garlic, and basil into the pot and continue to cook for four minutes.

2. Into the soup pot, add the crushed tomatoes, onion powder, thyme, nutritional yeast, and vegetable broth. Bring this mixture to a boil. Crack the lasagna noodles into small pieces and add them into the pot. Reduce the heat, fit on a lid, and allow the soup to simmer on low for twenty minutes.

3. Serve the soup topped with the vegan mozzarella shreds.

Nutrition:

Calories: 134

 Total fat: 9g

Saturated fat: 5g

Sodium: 118mg

Carbs: 19g

Fiber: 9g

Protein: 6g

Tabbouleh Salad

Preparation time: 5minutes

Cooking time: 12minutes

Servings: 4

Ingredients:

- 1/4 cup olive oil
- 2 tablespoons freshly squeezed lemon juice
- 2 garlic cloves, minced
- Pinch salt
- Pinch freshly ground black pepper
- 2 tomatoes, diced
- 1/2 cup chopped fresh parsley
- Cup dry bulgur wheat, cooked according to the package directions

Directions:

1. Merge together the olive oil, lemon juice, garlic, salt, and pepper. Gently stir in the tomatoes and parsley.

2. Attach the bulgur and toss to combine everything thoroughly. Taste and season with salt and pepper as needed.

Nutrition:

Calories: 110

Fats: 12.1g,

Carbs: 15.6g

Fiber: 7.5g

Sugar: 17.1g

Proteins: 7.6g

Sodium: 121mg

Caesar Salad

Preparation time: 10minutes

Cooking time: 0minutes

Servings: 4

Ingredients:

- 2 cups chopped romaine lettuce
- 2 tablespoons Caesar Dressing
- 1 serving Herbed Croutons or store-bought croutons
- Vegan cheese, grated (optional)
- Make it a meal
- 1/2 cup cooked pasta
- 1/2 cup canned chickpeas
- 2 additional tablespoons Caesar Dressing

Directions:

1. To make the Caesar salad
2. Merge together the lettuce, dressing, croutons, and cheese (if using).
3. To make it a meal
4. Add the pasta, chickpeas, and additional dressing. Toss to coat.

Nutrition:

Calories: 120

Fats: 13.1g,

Carbs: 12.6g

Fiber: 7.5g

Sugar: 17.1g

Proteins: 7.6g

Sodium: 121mg

Greek Potato Salad

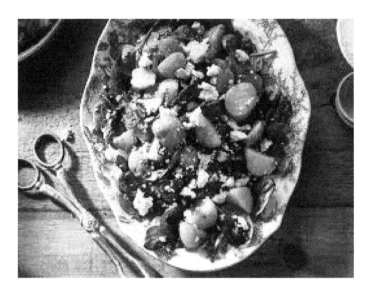

Preparation time: 10minutes

Cooking time: 20minutes

Servings: 3

Ingredients:

- 6 potatoes, scrubbed or peeled and chopped

- Salt

- 1/4 cup olive oil

- 2 tablespoons apple cider vinegar

- 2 tablespoons freshly squeezed lemon juice

- 1 teaspoon dried herbs

- 1/2 cucumber, chopped

- 1/4 red onion, diced

- 1/4 cup chopped pitted black olives

- Freshly ground black pepper

Directions:

1. Set the potatoes in a pot, add a pinch of salt, and pour in enough water to cover. Boil the water. Cook the potatoes for 15 to 20 minutes, until soft. Drain and set aside to cool. (Alternatively, put the potatoes in a large microwave-safe dish with a bit of water. Cover and heat on high power for 10 minutes.)

2. In a large bowl, whisk together the olive oil, vinegar, lemon juice, and dried herbs. Toss the cucumber, red onion, and olives with the dressing.

3. Add the cooked, cooled potatoes, and toss to combine. Taste and season with salt and pepper as needed.

Nutrition:

Calories: 110

Fats: 17.1g,

Carbs: 19.6g

Fiber: 7.5g

Sugar: 17.1g

Proteins: 7.6g

Sodium: 121mg

Pesto and White Bean Pasta Salad

Preparation time: 15minutes

Cooking time: 10minutes

Servings: 4

Ingredients:

- 1.1/2 cups canned cannellini beans

- 1/2 cup Spinach Pesto

- 1 cup chopped tomato or red bell pepper

- 1/4 red onion, finely diced

- 1/2 cup chopped pitted black olives

Directions:

1. In a large bowl, combine the pasta, beans, and pesto. Toss to combine.

2. Add the tomato, red onion, and olives, tossing thoroughly.

Nutrition:

Calories: 110

Fats: 17.1g,

Carbs: 19.6g

Fiber: 7.5g

Sugar: 17.1g

Proteins: 7.6g

Sodium: 121mg

Mediterranean Orzo and Chickpea Salad

Preparation time: 15minutes

Cooking time: 8minutes

Servings: 4

Ingredients:

- 1/4 cup olive oil
- 2 tablespoons freshly squeezed lemon juice
- Pinch salt
- 1.1/2 cups canned chickpeas, drained and rinsed
- 2 cups orzo or other small pasta shape, cooked according to the package directions, drained, and rinsed with cold water to cool
- 2 cups raw spinach, finely chopped
- 1 cup chopped cucumber
- 1/4 red onion, finely diced

Directions:

1. In a large bowl, whisk together the olive oil, lemon juice, and salt. Add the chickpeas and cooked orzo, and toss to coat.
2. Stir in the spinach, cucumber, and red onion.

Nutrition:

Calories: 110

Fats: 17.1g,

Carbs: 19.6g

Fiber: 7.5g

Sugar: 17.1g

Proteins: 7.6g

Sodium: 121mg

Vegetable Stir-Fry

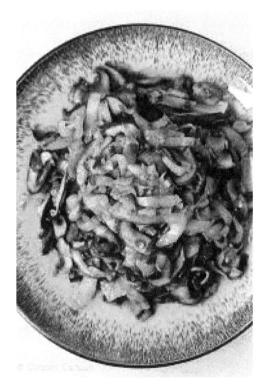

Preparation Time: 10minutes

Cooking time: 15minutes

Servings: 4

Ingredients:

- Zucchini (.50)

- Red Bell Pepper (.50)

- Broccoli (.50)

- Red Cabbage (1 C.)

- Brown Rice (.50 C.)

- Tamari Sauce (2 T.)

- Red Chili Pepper (1)

- Fresh Parsley (.25 t.)

- Garlic (4)

- Olive Oil (2 T.)

- Optional: Sesame Seeds

Directions:

1. To begin, you will want to cook your brown rice according to the directions that are placed on the package. Once this step is done, place the brown rice in a bowl and put it to the side.

2. Next, you will want to take a frying pan and place some water in the bottom. Bring the pan over medium heat and then add in your chopped vegetables. Once in place, cook the vegetables for five minutes or until they are tender.

3. When the vegetables are cooked through, you will then want to add in the parsley, cayenne powder, and the garlic. You will want to cook this mixture for a minute or so. Be sure you stir the ingredients so that nothing sticks to the bottom of your pan.

4. Now, add in the rice and tamari to your pan. You will cook this mixture for a few more minutes or until everything is warmed through.

5. For extra flavor, try adding sesame seeds before you enjoy your lunch! If you have any left-overs, you can keep this stir-fry in a sealed container for about five days in your fridge.

Nutrition:

Calories: 280

Protein: 10g

Fat: 12g

Carbs: 38g

Fibers: 6g

Chapter 5.   Dessert

Tart Apple Granita

Preparation time: 15 minutes, plus 4 hours freezing time

Cooking time: 0

Servings: 4

Ingredients:

- ½ cup granulated sugar
- ½ cup of water
- 2 cups unsweetened apple juice
- ¼ cup freshly squeezed lemon juice

Directions:

1. In a small saucepan over medium-high heat, heat the sugar and water.
2. Bring the mixture to a boil and then reduce the heat to low. Let it simmer for about 15 minutes or until the liquid has reduced by half.
3. Remove the pan from the heat and pour the liquid into a large shallow metal pan.
4. Let the liquid cool for about 30 minutes, and then stir in the apple juice and lemon juice.
5. Place the pan in the freezer.
6. After 1 hour, run a fork through the liquid to break up any ice crystals that have formed. Scrape down the sides as well.
7. Place the pan back in the freezer and repeat the stirring and scraping every 20 minutes, creating slush.
8. Serve when the mixture is completely frozen and looks like crushed ice, after about 3 hours.

Nutrition:

Calories: 157;

Fat: 0g;

Carbohydrates: 0g;

Phosphorus: 10mg;

Potassium: 141mg;

Sodium: 5mg;

Protein: 0g

Lemon-Lime Sherbet

Preparation time: 5 minutes, plus 3 hours chilling time

Cooking time: 15 minutes

Servings: 2

Ingredients:

- 2 cups of water
- 1 cup granulated sugar
- 3 tablespoons lemon zest, divided
- ½ cup freshly squeezed lemon juice
- Zest of 1 lime
- Juice of 1 lime
- ½ cup heavy (whipping) cream

Directions:

1. Place a large saucepan over medium-high heat and add the water, sugar, and two tablespoons of the lemon zest.

2. Bring the mixture to a boil and then reduce the heat and simmer for 15 minutes.

3. Transfer the mixture to a large bowl and add the remaining 1 tablespoon lemon zest, the lemon juice, lime zest, and lime juice.

4. Chill the mixture in the fridge until completely cold, about 3 hours.

5. Whisk in the heavy cream and transfer the mixture to an ice cream maker.

6. Freeze according to the manufacturer's instructions.

Nutrition:

Calories: 151;

Fat: 6g;

Carbohydrates: 26g;

Phosphorus: 10mg;

Potassium: 27mg;

Sodium: 6mg;

Protein: 0g

Tropical Vanilla Snow Cone

Preparation time: 15 minutes, plus freezing time

Cooking time: 0 minutes

Servings: 2

ingredients:

- 1 cup pineapple
- 1 cup of frozen strawberries
- 6 tablespoons water
- 2 tablespoons granulated sugar
- 1 tablespoon vanilla extract

Directions:

1. In a large saucepan, mix together the peaches, pineapple, strawberries, water, and sugar over medium-high heat and bring to a boil.
2. Reduce the heat to low and simmer the mixture, occasionally stirring, for 15 minutes.
3. Remove from the heat and let the mixture cool completely, for about 1 hour.
4. Stir in the vanilla and transfer the fruit mixture to a food processor or blender.
5. Purée until smooth, and pour the purée into a 9-by-13-inch glass baking dish.
6. Cover and place the dish in the freezer overnight.
7. When the fruit mixture is completely frozen, use a fork to scrape the sorbet until you have flaked flavored ice.
8. Scoop the ice flakes into four serving dishes.

Nutrition:

Calories: 92;

Fat: 0g;

Carbohydrates: 22g;

Phosphorus: 17mg;

Potassium: 145mg;

Sodium: 4mg;

Protein: 1g

Peanut Butter, Nut, And Fruit Cookies

Preparation time: 30 minutes

Cooking time: 0 minutes

Servings: 25

Ingredients:

- ¾ cup rolled oats

- ¼ cup chopped peanuts

- ½ cup coconut flakes, unsweetened

- ¼ cup and 2 tablespoons chopped cranberries, dried

- ¼ cup sliced almonds

- ¼ cup and 2 tablespoons raisins

- ¼ cup maple syrup

- ¾ cup peanut butter

Directions:

1. Take a baking sheet, line it with wax paper, and then set it aside until required.

2. Take a large bowl, place oats, almonds, and coconut flakes in it, add ¼ cup each of cranberries and raisins, and then stir until combined.

3. Add maple syrup and peanut butter, stir until well combined, and then scoop the mixture on the prepared baking sheet with some distance between them.

4. Flatten each scoop of cookie mixture slightly, press remaining cranberries and raisins into each cookie, and then let it chill for 20 minutes until firm.

5. Serve straight away.

Nutrition:

Calories: 140 Cal;

Fat: 7 g;

Protein: 3 g;

Carbs: 18 g;

Fiber: 5 g

Chocolate Covered Dates

Preparation time: 10 minutes

Cooking time: 3 minutes

Servings: 8

Ingredients:

- 16 medjool dates, pitted
- ½ teaspoon of sea salt
- ¾ cup almonds
- 1 teaspoon coconut oil
- 8 ounces chocolate chips, vegan

Directions:

1. Take a medium baking sheet, line it with parchment paper, and then set aside until required.
2. Place an almond into the pit of each date and then wrap the date tightly around it.
3. Place chocolate chips in a heatproof bowl, add oil, and then microwave for 2 to 3 minutes until chocolate melts, stirring every minute.
4. Working on one date at a time, dip each date into the chocolate mixture and then place it onto the prepared baking sheet.
5. Sprinkle salt over the prepared dates and then let them rest in the refrigerator for 1 hour until chocolate is firm.
6. Serve straight away.

Nutrition:

Calories: 179 Cal;

Fat: 7.7 g;

Protein: 3 g;

Carbs: 28.5 g;

Fiber: 3 g

Hot Chocolate

Preparation time: 5 minutes

Cooking time: 10 minutes

Servings: 4

Ingredients:

- ¼ cup of cocoa powder

- 1/8 teaspoon salt

- ½ teaspoon vanilla extract, unsweetened

- ¼ cup of coconut sugar

- 3 cups almond milk, unsweetened

Directions:

1. Take a medium saucepan, add salt, sugar, and cocoa powder in it, whisk until combined, and then whisk in milk.

2. Place the pan over medium-high heat and then bring the milk mixture to a simmer and turn hot, continue whisking.

3. Divide the hot chocolate evenly into four mugs and then serve.

Nutrition:

Calories: 137 Cal;

Fat: 3 g;

Protein: 6 g;

Carbs: 21 g;

Fiber: 2 g

Vanilla Cupcakes

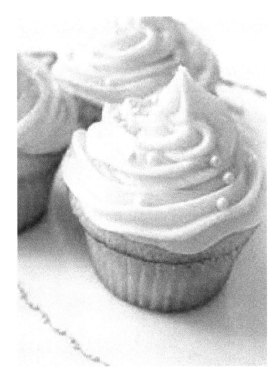

Preparation time: 10 minutes

Cooking time: 20 minutes

Servings: 18

Ingredients:

- 2 cups white whole-wheat flour

- 1 cup of coconut sugar

- ½ teaspoon salt

- 2 teaspoons baking powder

- 1 ¼ teaspoons vanilla extract, unsweetened

- ½ teaspoon baking soda

- 1 tablespoon apple cider vinegar

- ½ cup coconut oil, melted

- 1 ½ cups almond milk, unsweetened

Directions:

1. Switch on the oven, then set it to 350 degrees f, and then let it preheat.

2. Meanwhile, take a medium bowl, place vinegar in it, stir in milk, and then let it stand for 5 minutes until curdled.

3. Take a large bowl, place flour in it, add salt, baking soda and powder, and sugar and then stir until mixed.

4. Take a separate large bowl, pour in curdled milk mixture, add vanilla and coconut oil and then whisk until combined.

5. Whisk almond milk mixture into the flour mixture until smooth batter comes together, and then spoon the mixture into two 12-cups muffin pans lined with muffin cups.

6. Bake the muffins for 15 to 20 minutes until firm and the top turn golden brown, and then let them cool on the wire rack completely.

7. Serve straight away.

Nutrition:

Calories: 152.4 Cal;

Fat: 6.4 g;

Protein: 1.5 g;

Carbs: 22.6 g;

Fiber: 0.5 g

Garlic and Herb Oodles

Preparation Time: 5minutes

Cooking time: 2minutes

Servings: 3

Ingredients:

- 1 teaspoon extra-virgin olive oil or 2 tablespoons vegetable broth

- 1 teaspoon minced garlic (about 1 clove)

- 4 medium zucchinis, spiraled

- 1/2 teaspoon dried basil

- 1/2 teaspoon dried oregano

- 1/41/4 to 1/2 teaspoon red pepper flakes, to taste

- 1/4 teaspoon salt (optional)

- 1/4 teaspoon freshly ground black pepper

Directions:

1. Heat the olive oil. Add the garlic, zucchini, basil, oregano, red pepper flakes, salt (if using), and black pepper. Sauté for 1 to 2 minutes, until barely tender.

2. Divide the oodles evenly among 4 storage containers. Let cool before sealing the lids.

Nutrition:

Calories: 120

Protein: 10g

Fat: 44g

Carbs: 32g

Fibers: 5g

Stuffed Dried Figs

Preparation time: 20 minutes

Cooking time: 0 minutes

Servings: 4

Ingredients:

- 12 dried figs
- 2 tbsps. Thyme honey
- 2 tbsps. Sesame seeds
- 24 walnut halves

Directions:

1. Cut off the tough stalk ends of the figs.
2. Slice open each fig.
3. Stuff the fig openings with two walnut halves and close
4. Arrange the figs on a plate, drizzle with honey, and sprinkle the sesame seeds on it.
5. Serve.

Nutrition:

Calories: 110kcal

Carbs: 26

Fat: 3g,

Protein: 1g

Feta Cheesecake

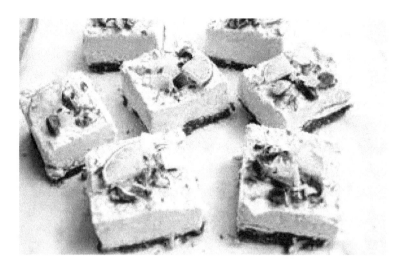

Preparation time: 30 minutes

Cooking time: 90 minutes

Servings: 12

Ingredients:

- 2 cups graham cracker crumbs (about 30 crackers)
- ½ tsp ground cinnamon
- 6 tbsps. Unsalted butter, melted
- ½ cup sesame seeds, toasted
- 12 ounces cream cheese, softened
- 1 cup crumbled feta cheese
- 1 cup of sugar
- 2 cups plain yogurt
- 2 tbsps. Grated lemon zest
- 1 tsp vanilla

Directions:

1. Set the oven to 350°f.

2. Mix the cracker crumbs, butter, cinnamon, and sesame seeds with a fork. Move the combination to a springform pan and spread until it is even. Refrigerate.

3. In a separate bowl, mix the cream cheese and feta. With an electric mixer, beat both kinds of cheese together., beating the mixture with each new addition. Add sugar, then keep beating until creamy. Mix in yogurt, vanilla, and lemon zest.

4. Bring out the refrigerated springform and spread the batter on it. Then place it in a baking pan. Pour water in the pan till it is halfway full.

5. Bake for about 50 minutes. Remove cheesecake and allow it to cool. Refrigerate for at least 4 hours.

6. It is done. Serve when ready.

Nutrition:

Calories: 98kcal

Carbs: 7g

Fat: 7g

Protein: 3g

Melomakarona

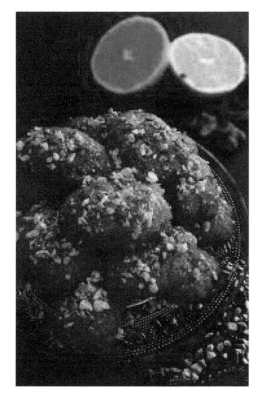

Preparation time: 20 minutes

Cooking time: 45 minutes

Servings: 20

Ingredients:

- 4 cups of sugar, divided

- 4 cups of water

- 1 cup plus 1 tbsp. Honey, divided

- 1 (2-inch) strip orange peel, pith removed

- 1 cinnamon stick

- ½ cup extra-virgin olive oil

- ¼ cup unsalted butter,

- ¼ cup metaxa brandy or any other brandy

- 1 tbsp. Grated

- Orange zest

- ¾ cup of orange juice

- ¼ tsp baking soda

- 3 cups pastry flour

- ¾ cup fine semolina flour

- 1 ½ tsp baking powder

- 4 tsp ground cinnamon, divided

- 1 tsp ground cloves, divided

- 1 cup finely chopped walnut

- 1/3 cup brown sugar

Directions:

1. Mix 3 ½ cups of sugar, 1 cup honey, orange peel, cinnamon stick, and water in a pot and heat it for about 10 minutes.

2. Mix the sugar, oil, and butter for about minutes, then add the brandy, leftover honey, and zest. Then add a mixture of baking soda and orange juice. Mix thoroughly.

3. In a distinct bowl, blend the pastry flour, baking powder, semolina, 2 tsp of cinnamon, and ½ tsp. Of cloves. Add the mixture to the mixer slowly. Run the mixer until the ingredients form a dough. Cover and set aside for 30 minutes.

4. Set the oven to 350°f

5. With your palms, form small oval balls from the dough. Make a total of forty balls.

6. Bake the cookie balls for 30 minutes, then drop them in the prepared syrup.

7. Create a mixture with the walnuts, leftover cinnamon, and cloves. Spread the mixture on the top of the baked cookies.

8. Serve the cookies or store them in a closed-lid container.

Nutrition:

Calories: 294kcal

Carbs: 44g

Fat: 12g

Protein: 3g

Loukoumades (Fried Honey Balls)

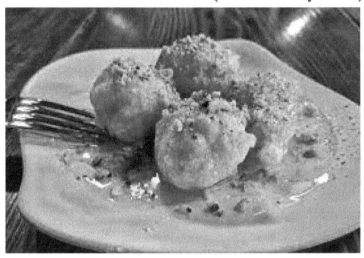

Preparation time: 20 minutes

Cooking time: 45 minutes

Servings: 10

Ingredients:

- 2 cups of sugar
- 1 cup of water
- 1 cup honey
- 1 ½ cups tepid water
- 1 tbsp. Brown sugar
- ¼ cup of vegetable oil
- 1 tbsp. Active dry yeast
- 1 ½ cups all-purpose flour, 1 cup cornstarch, ½ tsp salt
- Vegetable oil for frying
- 1 ½ cups chopped walnuts
- ¼ cup ground cinnamon

Directions:

1. Boil the sugar and water on medium heat. Add honey after 10 minutes. Cool and set aside.

2. Mix the tepid water, oil, brown sugar,' and yeast in a large bowl. Allow it to sit for 10 minutes. In a distinct bowl, blend the flour, salt, and cornstarch. With your hands mix the yeast and the flour to make a wet dough. Cover and set aside for 2 hours.

3. Fry in oil at 350°f. Use your palm to measure the sizes of the dough as they are dropped in the frying pan. Fry each batch for about 3-4 minutes.

4. Immediately the loukoumades are done frying, drop them in the prepared syrup.

5. Serve with cinnamon and walnuts.

Nutrition:

Calories: 355kcal

Carbs: 64g

Fat: 7g

Protein: 6g

Raspberry Muffins

Preparation time: 10 minutes

Cooking time: 25 minutes

Servings: 12

Ingredients:

- ½ cup and 2 tablespoons whole-wheat flour
- 1 ½ cup raspberries, fresh and more for decorating
- 1 cup white whole-wheat flour
- 1/8 teaspoon salt
- ¾ cup of coconut sugar
- 2 teaspoons baking powder
- 1 teaspoon apple cider vinegar
- 1 ¼ cups water
- ½ cup olive oil

Directions:

1. Switch on the oven, then set it to 400 degrees f and let it preheat.
2. Meanwhile, take a large bowl, place both flours in it, add salt and baking powder and then stir until combined.
3. Take a medium bowl, add oil to it, and then whisk in the sugar until dissolved.
4. Whisk in vinegar and water until blended, slowly stir in flour mixture until smooth batter comes together, and then fold in berries.
5. Take a 12-cups muffin pan, grease it with oil, fill evenly with the prepared mixture and then put a raspberry on top of each muffin.
6. Bake the muffins for 25 minutes until the top golden brown, and then serve.

Nutrition:

Calories: 109 Cal;

Fat: 3.4 g;

Protein: 2.1 g;

Carbs: 17.6 g;

Chocolate Chip Cake

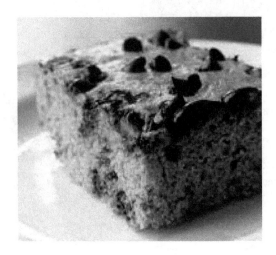

Preparation time: 10 minutes

Cooking time: 50 minutes

Servings: 10

Ingredients:

- 2 cups white whole-wheat flour

- ¼ teaspoon baking soda

- 1/3 cup coconut sugar

- 2 teaspoons baking powder

- ½ teaspoon salt

- ½ cup chocolate chips, vegan

- 1 teaspoon vanilla extract, unsweetened

- 1 tablespoon applesauce

- 1 teaspoon apple cider vinegar

- ¼ cup melted coconut oil

- ½ teaspoon almond extract, unsweetened

- 1 cup almond milk, unsweetened

Directions:

1. Switch on the oven, then set it to 360 degrees f and let it preheat.

2. Meanwhile, take a 9-by-5 inches loaf pan, grease it with oil, and then set aside until required.

3. Take a large bowl, add sugar to it, pour in oil, vanilla and almond extract, vinegar, apple sauce, and milk, and then whisk until well combined.

4. Take a large bowl, place flour in it, add salt, baking powder, and soda, and then stir until mixed.

5. Stir the flour mixture into the milk mixture until smooth batter comes together, and then fold in 1/3 cup of chocolate chips.

6. Spoon the batter into the loaf pan, scatter remaining chocolate chips on top and then bake for 50 minutes.

7. When done, let the bread cool for 10 minutes and then cut it into slices.

8. Serve straight away.

Nutrition:

Calories: 218 Cal;

Fat: 8 g;

Protein: 3.4 g;

Carbs: 32 g;

Fiber: 2 g

Coffee Cake

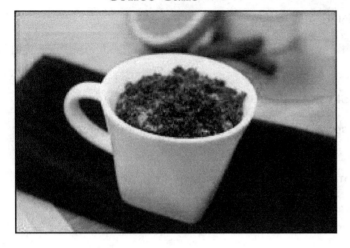

Preparation time: 10 minutes

Cooking time: 45 minutes

Servings: 9

Ingredients:

For the cake:

- 1/3 cup coconut sugar
- 1 teaspoon vanilla extract, unsweetened
- ¼ cup olive oil
- 1/8 teaspoon almond extract, unsweetened
- 1 ¾ cup white whole-wheat flour
- 2 teaspoons baking powder
- ½ teaspoon salt
- ¼ teaspoon baking soda
- 1 teaspoon apple cider vinegar
- 1 tablespoon applesauce
- 1 cup almond milk, unsweetened

For the streusel:

- ½ cup white whole-wheat flour

- 2 teaspoons cinnamon

- 1/3 cup coconut sugar

- ½ teaspoon salt

- 2 tablespoons olive oil

- 1 tablespoon coconut butter

Directions:

1. Switch on the oven, then set it to 350 degrees f and let it preheat.

2. Meanwhile, take a large bowl, pour in milk, add applesauce, vinegar, sugar, oil, vanilla, and almond extract and then whisk until blended.

3. Take a medium bowl, place flour in it, add salt, baking powder, and soda and then stir until mixed.

4. Stir the flour mixture into the milk mixture until smooth batter comes together, and then spoon the mixture into a loaf pan lined with parchment paper.

5. Prepare streusel and for this, take a medium bowl, place flour in it, and then add sugar, salt, and cinnamon.

6. Stir until mixed, and then mix butter and oil with fingers until the crumble mixture comes together.

7. Spread the prepared streusel on top of the batter of the cake and then bake for 45 minutes until the top turn golden brown and cake have thoroughly cooked.

8. When done, let the cake rest in its pan for 10 minutes, remove it to cool completely and then cut it into slices.

9. Serve straight away.

Nutrition:

Calories: 259 Cal;

Fat: 10 g;

Protein: 3 g;

Carbs: 37 g;

Fiber: 1 g

Chocolate Marble Cake

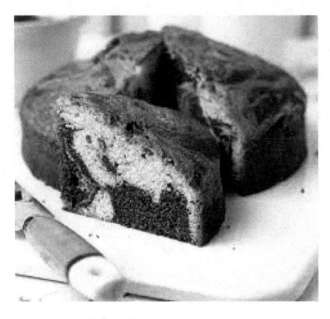

Preparation time: 15 minutes

Cooking time: 50 minutes

Servings: 8

Ingredients:

- 1 ½ cup white whole-wheat flour

- 1 tablespoon flaxseed meal

- 2 ½ tablespoons cocoa powder

- ¼ teaspoon salt

- 4 tablespoons chopped walnuts

- 1 teaspoon baking powder

- 2/3 cup coconut sugar

- ¼ teaspoon baking soda

- 1 teaspoon vanilla extract, unsweetened

- 3 tablespoons peanut butter

- ¼ cup olive oil

- 1 cup almond milk, unsweetened

Directions:

1. Switch on the oven, then set it to 350 degrees f and let it preheat.
2. Meanwhile, take a medium bowl, place flour in it, add salt, baking powder, and soda in it and then stir until mixed.
3. Take a large bowl, pour in milk, add sugar, flaxseed, oil, and vanilla, whisk until sugar has dissolved, and then whisk in flour mixture until smooth batter comes together.
4. Spoon half of the prepared batter in a medium bowl, add cocoa powder and then stir until combined.
5. Add peanut butter into the other bowl and then stir until combined.
6. Take a loaf pan, line it with a parchment sheet, spoon half of the chocolate batter in it, and then spread it evenly.
7. Layer the chocolate batter with half of the peanut butter batter, cover with the remaining chocolate batter and then layer with the remaining peanut butter batter.
8. Make swirls into the batter with a toothpick, smooth the top with a spatula, sprinkle walnuts on top, and then bake for 50 minutes until done.
9. When done, let the cake rest in its pan for 10 minutes, then remove it to cool completely and cut it into slices.
10. serve straight away.

Nutrition:

Calories: 299 Cal;

Fat: 14 g;

Protein: 6 g;

Carbs: 39 g;

Fiber: 3 g

Sweet Chocolate Cookies

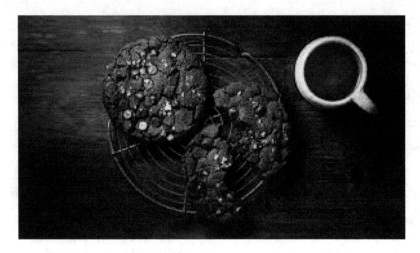

Preparation time: 10 minutes

Cooking time: 10 minutes

Servings: 11

Ingredients:

- 1 ¼ cups white whole-wheat flour

- 1 ½ tablespoon flax seeds

- ½ teaspoon baking soda

- ½ cup of coconut sugar

- ¼ teaspoon of sea salt

- ¼ cup powdered coconut sugar

- 1 teaspoon baking powder

- 2 teaspoons vanilla extract, unsweetened

- 4 ½ tablespoons water

- ½ cup of coconut oil

- 1 cup chocolate chips, vegan

Directions:

1. Take a large bowl, place flax seeds in it, stir in water and then let the mixture rest for 5 minutes until creamy.

2. Then add remaining ingredients into the flax seed's mixture except for flour and chocolate chips and then beat until light batter comes together.

3. Beat in flour, ¼ cup at a time, until smooth batter comes together, and then fold in chocolate chips.

4. Use an ice cream scoop to scoop the batter onto a baking sheet lined with parchment sheet with some distance between cookies and then bake for 10 minutes until cookies turn golden brown.

5. When done, let the cookies cool on the baking sheet for 3 minutes and then cool completely on the wire rack for 5 minutes.

6. Serve straight away.

Nutrition:

Calories: 141 Cal;

Fat: 7 g;

Protein: 1 g;

Carbs: 17 g;

Fiber: 2 g

Lemon Cake

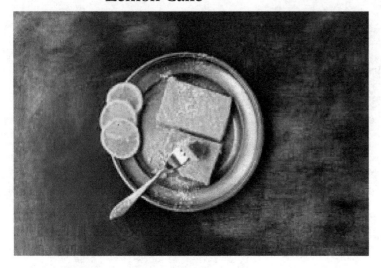

Preparation time: 10 minutes

Cooking time: 50 minutes

Servings: 9

Ingredients:

- 1 ½ cup white whole-wheat flour

- 1 ½ teaspoon baking powder

- 2 tablespoons almond flour

- 1 lemon, zested

- ¼ teaspoon baking soda

- 1/8 teaspoon turmeric powder

- 1/3 teaspoon salt

- ¼ teaspoon vanilla extract, unsweetened

- 1/3 cup lemon juice

- ½ cup maple syrup

- ¼ cup olive oil

- ¼ cup of water

For the frosting:

- 1 tablespoon lemon juice

- 1/8 teaspoon salt

- ¼ cup maple syrup

- 2 tablespoons powdered sugar

- 6 ounces vegan cream cheese, softened

Directions:

1. Switch on the oven, then set it to 350 degrees f and let it preheat.

2. Take a large bowl, pour in water, lemon juice, and oil, add vanilla extract and maple syrup, and whisk until blended.

3. Whisk in flour, ¼ cup at a time, until smooth, and then whisk in almond flour, salt, turmeric, lemon zest, baking soda, and powder until well combined.

4. Take a loaf pan, grease it with oil, spoon prepared batter in it, and then bake for 50 minutes.

5. Meanwhile, prepare the frosting and for this, take a small bowl, place all of its ingredients in it, whisk until smooth, and then let it chill until required.

6. When the cake has cooked, let it cool for 10 minutes in its pan and then let it cool completely on the wire rack.

7. Spread the prepared frosting on top of the cake, slice the cake, and then serve.

Nutrition:

Calories: 275 Cal;

Fat: 12 g;

Protein: 3 g;

Carbs: 38 g;

Fiber: 1 g

Banana Muffins

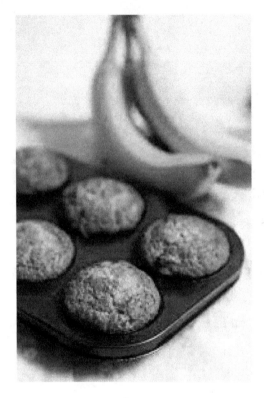

Preparation time: 10 minutes

Cooking time: 30 minutes

Servings: 12

Ingredients:

- 1 ½ cups mashed banana

- 1 ½ cups and 2 tablespoons white whole-wheat flour, divided

- ¼ cup of coconut sugar

- ¾ cup rolled oats, divided

- 1 teaspoon ginger powder

- 1 tablespoon ground cinnamon, divided

- 2 teaspoons baking powder

- ½ teaspoon salt

- 1 teaspoon baking soda

- 1 tablespoon vanilla extract, unsweetened

- ½ cup maple syrup

- 1 tablespoon rum

- ½ cup of coconut oil

Directions:

1. Switch on the oven, then set it to 350 degrees f and let it preheat.

2. Meanwhile, take a medium bowl, place 1 ½ cup flour in it, add ½ cup oars, ginger, baking powder and soda, salt, and 2 teaspoons cinnamon and then stir until mixed.

3. Place ¼ cup of coconut oil in a heatproof bowl, melt it in the microwave oven and then whisk in maple syrup until combined.

4. Add mashed banana along with rum and vanilla, stir until combined, and then whisk this mixture into the flour mixture until smooth batter comes together.

5. Take a separate medium bowl, place remaining oats and flour in it, add cinnamon, coconut sugar, and coconut oil and then stir with a fork until crumbly mixture comes together.

6. Take a 12-cups muffin pan, fill evenly with prepared batter, top with oats mixture, and then bake for 30 minutes until firm and the top turn golden brown.

7. When done, let the muffins cool for 5 minutes in its pan and then cool the muffins completely before serving.

Nutrition:

Calories: 240 Cal;

Fat: 9.3 g;

Protein: 2.6 g;

Carbs: 35.4 g;

Fiber: 2 g

No-Bake Cookies

Preparation time: 30 minutes

Cooking time: 0 minutes

Servings: 9

Ingredients:

- 1 cup rolled oats
- ¼ cup of cocoa powder
- 1/8 teaspoon salt
- 1 teaspoon vanilla extract, unsweetened
- ¼ cup and 2 tablespoons peanut butter, divided
- 6 tablespoons coconut oil, divided
- ¼ cup and 1 tablespoon maple syrup, divided

Directions:

1. Take a small saucepan, place it over low heat, add 5 tablespoons of coconut oil and then let it melt.
2. Whisk in 2 tablespoons peanut butter, salt, 1 teaspoon vanilla extract, and ¼ cup each of cocoa powder and maple syrup, and then whisk until well combined.
3. Remove pan from heat, stir in oats and then spoon the mixture evenly into 9 cups of a muffin pan.
4. Wipe clean the pan, return it over low heat, add remaining coconut oil, maple syrup, and peanut butter, stir until combined, and then cook for 2 minutes until thoroughly warmed.
5. Drizzle the peanut butter sauce over the oat mixture in the muffin pan and then let it freeze for 20 minutes or more until set.
6. Serve straight away.

Nutrition:

Calories: 213 Cal;

Fat: 14.8 g;

Protein: 4 g;

Carbs: 17.3 g;

Fiber: 2.1 g

Peanut Butter and Oat Bars

Preparation time: 40 minutes

Cooking time: 8 minutes

Servings: 8

Ingredients:

- 1 cup rolled oats
- 1/8 teaspoon salt
- ¼ cup chocolate chips, vegan
- ¼ cup maple syrup
- 1 cup peanut butter

Directions:

1. Take a medium saucepan, place it over medium heat, add peanut butter, salt, and maple syrup and then whisk until combined and thickened; this will take 5 minutes.
2. Remove pan from heat, place oats in a bowl, pour peanut butter mixture on it and then stir until well combined.
3. Take an 8-by-6 inches baking dish, line it with a parchment sheet, spoon the oats mixture in it, and then spread evenly, pressing the mixture into the dish.
4. Sprinkle the chocolate chips on top, press them into the bar mixture and then let the mixture rest in the refrigerator for 30 minutes or more until set.
5. When ready to eat, cut the bar mixture into even size pieces and then serve.

Nutrition:

Calories: 274 Cal;

Fat: 17 g;

Protein: 10 g;

Carbs: 19 g;

Fiber: 3 g

Baked Apples

Preparation time: 5 minutes

Cooking time: 20 minutes

Servings: 4

Ingredients:

- 6 medium apples, peeled, cut into chunks
- 1 teaspoon ground cinnamon
- 2 tablespoons melted coconut oil

Directions:

1. Switch on the oven, then set it to 350 degrees f and let it preheat.
2. Take a medium baking dish, and then spread apple pieces in it.
3. Take a small bowl, place coconut oil in it, stir in cinnamon, drizzle this mixture over apples and then toss until coated.
4. Place the baking dish into the oven and then bake for 20 minutes or more until apples turn soft, stirring halfway.
5. Serve straight away.

Nutrition:

Calories: 170 Cal;

Fat: 3.8 g;

Protein: 0.5 g;

Carbs: 31 g;

Fiber: 5.5 g

Chocolate Strawberry Shake

Preparation time: 5 minutes

Cooking time: 0 minutes

Servings: 2

Ingredients:

- 2 cups almond milk, unsweetened
- 4 bananas, peeled, frozen
- 4 tablespoons cocoa powder
- 2 cups strawberries, frozen

Directions:

1. Place all the ingredients into the jar of a high-speed food processor or blender in the order stated in the ingredients list and then cover it with the lid.
2. Pulse for 1 minute until smooth, and then serve.

Nutrition:

Calories: 208 Cal;

Fat: 0.2 g;

Protein: 12.4 g;

Carbs: 26.2 g;

Fiber: 1.4 g

Chocolate Clusters

Preparation time: 15 minutes

Cooking time: 0 minutes

Servings: 12

Ingredients:

- 1 cup chopped dark chocolate, vegan
- 1 cup cashews, roasted, salt
- 1 teaspoon sea salt flakes

Directions:

1. Take a large baking sheet, line it with wax paper, and then set aside until required.
2. Take a medium bowl, place chocolate in it, and then microwave for 1 minute.
3. Stir the chocolate and then continue microwaving it at 1-minute intervals until chocolate melts completely, stirring at every interval.
4. When melted, stir the chocolate to bring it to 90 degrees f and then stir in cashews.
5. Scoop the walnut-chocolate mixture on the prepared baking sheet, ½ tablespoons per cluster, and then sprinkle with salt.
6. Let the clusters stand at room temperature until harden and then serve.

Nutrition:

Calories: 79.4 Cal;

Fat: 6.6 g;

Protein: 1 g;

Carbs: 5.8 g;

Fiber: 1.1 g

Banana Coconut Cookies

Preparation time: 40 minutes

Cooking time: 0 minutes

Servings: 8

Ingredients:

- 1 ½ cup shredded coconut, unsweetened
- 1 cup mashed banana

Directions:

1. Switch on the oven, then set it to 350 degrees f and let it preheat.
2. Take a medium bowl, place the mashed banana in it and then stir in coconut until well combined.
3. Take a large baking sheet, line it with a parchment sheet, and then scoop the prepared mixture on it, 2 tablespoons of mixture per cookie.
4. Place the baking sheet into the refrigerator and then let it cool for 30 minutes or more until harden.
5. Serve straight away.

Nutrition:

Calories: 51 Cal;

Fat: 3 g;

Protein: 0.2 g;

Carbs: 4 g;

Fiber: 1 g

Chocolate Pots

Preparation time: 4 hours 10 minutes

Cooking time: 3 minutes

Servings: 4

Ingredients:

- 6 ounces chocolate, unsweetened
- 1 cup medjool dates, pitted
- 1 ¾ cups almond milk, unsweetened

Directions:

1. Cut the chocolate into small pieces, place them in a heatproof bowl and then microwave for 2 to 3 minutes until melt completely, stirring every minute.
2. Place dates in a blender, pour in the milk, and then pulse until smooth.
3. Add chocolate into the blender and then pulse until combined.
4. Divide the mixture into the small mason jars and then let them rest for 4 hours until set.
5. Serve straight away.

Nutrition:

Calories: 321 Cal;

Fat: 19 g;

Protein: 6 g;

Carbs: 34 g;

Fiber: 4 g

Maple and Tahini Fudge

Preparation time: 2 hours

Cooking time: 3 minutes

Servings: 15

Ingredients:

- 1 cup dark chocolate chips, vegan
- ¼ cup maple syrup
- ½ cup tahini

Directions:

1. Take a heatproof bowl, place chocolate chips in it and then microwave for 2 to 3 minutes until melt completely, stirring every minute.
2. When melted, remove the chocolate bowl from the oven and then whisk in maple syrup and tahini until smooth.
3. Take a 4-by-8 inches baking dish, line it with wax paper, spoon the chocolate mixture in it and then press it into the baking dish.
4. Cover with another sheet with wax paper, press it down until smooth, and then let the fudge rest for 1 hour in the freezer until set.
5. Then cut the fudge into 15 squares and serve.

Nutrition:

Calories: 110.7 Cal;

Fat: 5.3 g;

Protein: 2.2 g;

Carbs: 15.1 g;

Fiber: 1.6 g

Creaseless

Preparation time: 5 minutes

Cooking time: 0 minutes

Servings: 5

Ingredients:

- 3 tablespoons agave syrup
- 1 cup coconut milk, unsweetened
- ½ teaspoon vanilla extract, unsweetened
- 1 cup of orange juice

Directions:

1. Place all the ingredients in a food processor or blender and then pulse until combined.
2. Pour the mixture into five molds of popsicle pan, insert a stick into each mold and then let it freeze for a minimum of 4 hours until hard.
3. Serve when ready.

Nutrition:

Calories: 152 Cal;

Fat: 10 g;

Protein: 1 g;

Carbs: 16 g;

Fiber: 1 g

Almonds and Oats Pudding

Preparation time: 10 minutes

Cooking time: 15 minutes

Servings: 4

Ingredients:

- 1 tablespoon lemon juice
- Zest of 1 lime
- 1 and ½ cups of almond milk
- 1 teaspoon almond extract
- ½ cup oats
- 2 tablespoons stevia
- ½ cup silver almonds, chopped

Directions:

1. In a pan, blend the almond milk plus the lime zest and the other ingredients, whisk, bring to a simmer and cook over medium heat for 15 minutes.
2. Split the mix into bowls then serve cold.

Nutrition:

Calories 174

Fat 12.1

Fiber 3.2

Carbs 3.9

Protein 4.8

Chocolate Cups

Preparation time: 2 hours

Cooking time: 0 minutes

Servings: 6

Ingredients:

- ½ cup avocado oil

- 1 cup, chocolate, melted

- 1 teaspoon matcha powder

- 3 tablespoons stevia

Directions:

1. In a bowl, mix the chocolate with the oil and the rest of the ingredients.
2. Whisk well and divide into cups.
3. Keep in the freezer for 2 hours before serving.

Nutrition:

Calories 174

Fat 9.1

Fiber 2.2

Carbs 3.9

Protein 2.8

Mango Bowls

Preparation time: 30 minutes

Cooking time: 0 minutes

Servings: 4

Ingredients:

- 3 cups mango, cut into medium chunks

- ½ cup of coconut water

- ¼ cup stevia

- 1 teaspoon vanilla extract

Directions:

1. In a blender, blend the mango plus the rest of the ingredients, pulse well.
2. Divide into bowls and serve cold.

Nutrition:

Calories 122

Fat 4

Fiber 5.3

Carbs 6.6

Protein 4.5

Cocoa and Pears Cream

Preparation time: 10 minutes

Cooking time: 0 minutes

Servings: 4

Ingredients:

- 2 cups heavy creamy
- 1/3 cup stevia
- ¾ cup cocoa powder
- 6 ounces dark chocolate, chopped
- Zest of 1 lemon
- 2 pears, chopped

Directions:

1. In a blender, blend the cream plus the stevia and the rest of the ingredients.
2. Blend well.
3. Divide into cups and serve cold.

Nutrition:

Calories 172

Fat 5.6

Fiber 3.5

Carbs 7.6

Protein 4

Pineapple Pudding

Preparation time: 10 minutes

Cooking time: 40 minutes

Servings: 4

Ingredients:

- 3 cups almond flour
- ¼ cup olive oil
- 1 teaspoon vanilla extract
- 2 and ¼ cups stevia
- 1 and ¼ cup natural apple sauce
- 2 teaspoons baking powder
- 1 and ¼ cups of almond milk
- 2 cups pineapple, chopped
- Cooking spray

Directions:

1. In a bowl, blend the almond flour plus the oil and the rest of the ingredients except the cooking spray and stir well.
2. Grease a cake pan with the cooking spray, pour the pudding mix inside, introduce in the oven and bake at 370 degrees f for 40 minutes.
3. Serve the pudding cold.

Nutrition:

Calories 223

Fat 8.1

Fiber 3.4

Carbs 7.6

Protein 3.4

Lime Vanilla Fudge

Preparation time: 3 hours

Cooking time: 0 minutes

Servings: 6

Ingredients:

- 1/3 cup cashew butter
- 5 tablespoons lime juice
- ½ teaspoon lime zest, grated
- 1 tablespoons stevia

Directions:

1. In a bowl, mix the cashew butter with the other ingredients and whisk well.
2. Line a muffin tray with parchment paper, scoop 1 tablespoon of lime fudge mix in each of the muffin tins and keep in the freezer for 3 hours before serving.

Nutrition:

Calories 200

Fat 4.5

Fiber 3.4

Carbs 13.5

Protein 5

Mixed Berries Stew

Preparation time: 10 minutes

Cooking time: 15 minutes

Servings: 6

Ingredients:

- Zest of 1 lemon, grated
- Juice of 1 lemon
- ½ pint blueberries
- 1-pint strawberries halved
- 2 cups of water
- 2 tablespoons stevia

Directions:

1. In a pan, blend the berries plus the water, stevia and the other ingredients.
2. Bring to a simmer, cook over medium heat for 15 minutes.
3. Divide into bowls and serve cold.

Nutrition:

Calories 172

Fat 7

Fiber 3.4

Carbs 8

Protein 2.3

Orange and Apricots Cake

Preparation time: 10 minutes

Cooking time: 20 minutes

Servings: 8

Ingredients:

- ¾ cup stevia
- 2 cups almond flour
- ¼ cup olive oil
- ½ cup almond milk
- 1 teaspoon baking powder
- ½ teaspoon vanilla extract
- Juice and zest of 2 oranges
- 2 cups apricots, chopped

Directions:

1. In a bowl, blend the stevia plus the flour and the rest of the ingredients, whisk and pour into a cake pan lined with parchment paper.
2. Introduce in the oven at 375 degrees f, bake for 20 minutes.
3. Cool down, slice and serve.

Nutrition:

Calories 221

Fat 8.3

Fiber 3.4

Carbs 14.5

Protein 5

Blueberry Cake

Preparation time: 10 minutes

Cooking time: 30 minutes

Servings: 6

Ingredients:

- 2 cups almond flour
- 3 cups blueberries
- 1 cup walnuts, chopped
- 3 tablespoons stevia
- 1 teaspoon vanilla extract
- 2 tablespoons avocado oil
- 1 teaspoon baking powder
- Cooking spray

Directions:

1. In a bowl, blend the flour plus the blueberries, walnuts and the other ingredients except for the cooking spray, and stir well.
2. Grease a cake pan with the cooking spray, pour the cake mix inside, introduce everything in the oven at 350 degrees f and bake for 30 minutes.
3. Cool the cake down, slice and serve.

Nutrition:

Calories 225

Fat 9

Fiber 4.5

Carbs 10.2

Protein 4.5

Almond Peaches Mix

Preparation time: 10 minutes

Cooking time: 10 minutes

Servings: 4

Ingredients:

- 1/3 cup almonds, toasted
- 1/3 cup pistachios, toasted
- 1 teaspoon mint, chopped
- ½ cup of coconut water
- 1 teaspoon lemon zest, grated
- 4 peaches, halved
- 2 tablespoons stevia

Directions:

1. In a pan, combine the peaches with the stevia and the rest of the ingredients.
2. Simmer over medium heat for 10 minutes.
3. Divide into bowls and serve cold.

Nutrition:

Calories 135

Fat 4.1

Fiber 3.8

Carbs 4.1

Protein 2.3

Spiced Peaches

Preparation time: 5 minutes

Cooking time: 10 minutes

Servings: 2

Ingredients:

- Canned peaches with juices – 1 cup
- Cornstarch – ½ tsp.
- Ground cloves – 1 tsp.
- Ground cinnamon – 1 tsp.
- Ground nutmeg – 1 tsp.
- Zest of ½ lemon
- Water – ½ cup

Directions:

1. Drain peaches.
2. Combine cinnamon, cornstarch, nutmeg, ground cloves, and lemon zest in a pan on the stove.
3. Heat on medium heat and add peaches.
4. Bring to a boil, decrease the heat then simmer for 10 minutes.
5. Serve.

Nutrition:

Calories: 70;

Fat: 0g;

Carb: 14g;

Phosphorus: 23mg;

Potassium: 176mg;

Sodium: 3mg;

Protein: 1g

Pumpkin Cheesecake Bar

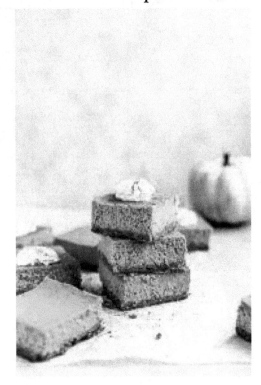

Preparation time: 10 minutes

Cooking time: 50 minutes

Servings: 4

Ingredients:

- Unsalted butter – 2 ½ tbsps.

- Cream cheese – 4 oz.

- All-purpose white flour – ½ cup

- Golden brown sugar – 3 tbsps.

- Granulated sugar – ¼ cup

- Pureed pumpkin – ½ cup

- Ground cinnamon – 1 tsp.

- Ground nutmeg – 1 tsp.

- Vanilla extract – 1 tsp.

Directions:

1. Preheat the oven to 350f.
2. Mix brown sugar and flour in a container.
3. Mix in the butter to form 'breadcrumbs.'
4. Place ¾ of this mixture in a dish.
5. Bake in the oven for 15 minutes. Remove and cool.
6. Lightly whisk the cream cheese, sugar, pumpkin, cinnamon, nutmeg, and vanilla until smooth.
7. Pour this mixture over the oven-baked base and sprinkle with the rest of the breadcrumbs from earlier.
8. Bake for 30 to 35 minutes more.
9. Cool, slice, and serve.

Nutrition:

Calories: 248;

Fat: 13g;

Carb: 33g;

Phosphorus: 67mg;

Potassium: 96mg;

Sodium: 146mg;

Protein: 4g

Blueberry Mini Muffins

Preparation time: 10 minutes

Cooking time: 35 minutes

Servings: 4

Ingredients:

- All-purpose white flour – ¼ cup
- Coconut flour – 1 tbsp.
- Baking soda – 1 tsp.
- Nutmeg – 1 tbsp. Grated
- Vanilla extract – 1 tsp.
- Stevia – 1 tsp.
- Fresh blueberries – ¼ cup

Directions:

1. Preheat the oven to 325f.
2. Mix all the ingredients in a bowl.
3. Divide the batter into four and spoon into a lightly oiled muffin tin.
4. Bake in the oven for 15 to 20 minutes or until cooked through.
5. Cool and serve.

Nutrition:

Calories: 62;

Fat: 0g;

Carb: 9g;

Phosphorus: 103mg;

Potassium: 65mg;

Sodium: 62mg;

Protein: 4g;

Baked Peaches with Cream Cheese

Preparation time: 10 minutes

Cooking time: 15 minutes

Servings: 4

Ingredients:

- Plain cream cheese – 1 cup
- Crushed meringue cookies – ½ cup
- Ground cinnamon – ¼ tsp.
- Pinch ground nutmeg
- Canned peach halves – 8, in juice
- Honey – 2 tbsp.

Directions:

1. Preheat the oven to 350f.
2. Line a baking sheet with parchment paper. Set aside.
3. In a small bowl, stir together the meringue cookies, cream cheese, cinnamon, and nutmeg.
4. Spoon the cream cheese mixture evenly into the cavities in the peach halves.
5. Place the peaches on the baking sheet and bake for 15 minutes or until the fruit is soft and the cheese is melted.
6. Remove the peaches from the baking sheet onto plates.
7. Drizzle with honey and serve.

Nutrition:

Calories: 260;

Fat: 20;

Carb: 19g;

Phosphorus: 74mg;

Potassium: 198mg;

Sodium: 216mg;

Protein: 4g;

Strawberry Ice Cream

Preparation time: 5 minutes

Cooking time: 5 minutes

Servings: 3

Ingredients:

- Stevia – ½ cup

- Lemon juice – 1 tbsp.

- Non-dairy coffee creamer – ¾ cup

- Strawberries – 10 oz.

- Crushed ice – 1 cup

Directions:

1. Blend everything in a blender until smooth.
2. Freeze until frozen.
3. Serve.

Nutrition:

Calories: 94.4;

Fat: 6g;

Carb: 8.3g;

Phosphorus: 25mg;

Potassium: 108mg;

Sodium: 25mg;

Protein: 1.3g;

Raspberry Brule

Preparation time: 15 minutes

Cooking time: 1 minute

Servings: 4

Ingredients:

- Light sour cream – ½ cup
- Plain cream cheese – ½ cup
- Brown sugar – ¼ cup, divided
- Ground cinnamon – ¼ tsp.
- Fresh raspberries – 1 cup

Directions:

1. Preheat the oven to broil.
2. In a bowl, beat together the cream cheese, sour cream, 2 tbsp. Brown sugar and cinnamon for 4 minutes or until the mixture are very smooth and fluffy.
3. Evenly divide the raspberries among 4 (4-ounce) ramekins.
4. Spoon the cream cheese mixture over the berries and smooth the tops.
5. Sprinkle ½ tbsp. Brown sugar evenly over each ramekin.
6. Place the ramekins on a baking sheet and broil 4 inches from the heating element until the sugar is caramelized and golden brown.
7. Cool and serve.

Nutrition:

Calories: 188;

Fat: 13g;

Carb: 16g;

Phosphorus: 60mg;

Potassium: 158mg;

Sodium: 132mg;

Crazy Chocolate Cake

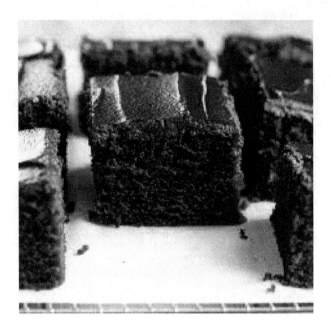

Preparation time: 15 minutes

Cooking time: 35 minutes

Servings: 12

Ingredients:

For the cake:

- Cooking spray, for greasing
- 1½ cups all-purpose flour
- 1 cup granulated sugar
- ¼ cup Dutch process cocoa powder
- 1 teaspoon baking soda
- ½ teaspoon salt
- 1 teaspoon white vinegar
- 5 tablespoons vegetable oil
- 1 teaspoon vanilla extract
- 1 cup water

For the frosting:

- 6 cups powdered sugar
- 1 cup cocoa powder
- 2 cups vegan butter, softened
- 1 teaspoon vanilla extract
- 1 pinch salt

Directions:

1. For the cake, warm your oven to 350°F. Grease or spray an 8-inch square baking dish or a 9-inch round cake pan.
2. In a large bowl, combine the flour, sugar, cocoa powder, baking soda, and salt. Add the vinegar, vegetable oil, vanilla extract, and water directly to the dry ingredients. Stir the batter until no lumps remain.
3. Put the batter into the greased dish and bake for 35 minutes or until a toothpick inserted into the center comes out clean.
4. Once the cake is baked, cool it in the pan for 10 minutes. Transfer it to a plate and refrigerate for about 30 minutes, then frost.
5. For the frosting, mix the powdered sugar plus cocoa powder in a large bowl. Beat the vegan butter on medium-high speed until pale and creamy using an electric hand mixer or a stand mixer with the paddle attachment.
6. Reduce the mixer speed to medium and add the powdered sugar and cocoa mix, ½ cup at a time, mixing well between each addition (about 5 minutes total). Add the vanilla extract and salt and mix on high speed for 1 minute.

Nutrition:

Calories: 831

Fat: 44 g

Carbs: 111 g

Protein: 5 g

Chunky Chocolate Peanut Butter Balls

Preparation time: 15 minutes

Cooking time: 0 minutes

Servings: 6

Ingredients:

- ½ cup crunchy peanut butter
- 1½ cups shredded coconut, divided
- 1 cup rolled oats
- ½ cup ground flaxseed
- ¼ cup chia seeds
- ½ cup dairy-free mini chocolate chips
- 1/3 cup maple syrup
- 1 teaspoon vanilla extract

Directions:

1. Melt the peanut butter in a microwave-safe dish for 15 to 20 seconds. In a large bowl, combine 1 cup of the shredded coconut, the rolled oats, ground flaxseed, chia seeds, and chocolate chips.
2. Pour in the melted peanut butter, maple syrup, and vanilla extract. Stir well to combine. Refrigerate within 15 to 20 minutes, until chilled enough that the mixture sticks together when pressed but not so cold that the peanut butter hardens.
3. Place the remaining ½ cup of shredded coconut into a shallow dish. Spoon out 2 tablespoons of the mixture at a time and roll into 1-inch balls.
4. Roll the balls in the remaining ½ cup of shredded coconut to coat. Refrigerate for up to a week.

Nutrition:

Calories: 528

Fat: 35 g

Carbs: 47 g

Protein: 12 g

Chocolate Peanut Butter Crispy Bars

Preparation time: 45 minutes

Cooking time: 0 minutes

Servings: 6-8

Ingredients:

- 1 cup dates
- 1 cup raw cashews
- ¼ cup Dutch process cocoa powder
- 1 teaspoon vanilla extract
- 1½ cups crunchy peanut butter
- 2 cups dairy-free chocolate chips
- 1 cup all-natural smooth peanut butter
- 3 cups puffed rice cereal

Directions:

1. Prepare an 8-inch square baking dish lined using parchment paper. Set aside. Soak the dates in a bowl of warm water for 10 minutes. Drain and pat dry.
2. In a food processor or blender, combine the dates, cashews, cocoa powder, and vanilla extract and process to form a thick dough.
3. Press into the baking dish. Cover with the crunchy peanut butter, spreading it into an even layer. Refrigerate for 5 minutes.
4. In a large microwave-safe bowl, combine the chocolate chips and smooth peanut butter. Microwave in 30-second increments, stirring in between, until smooth. Remove from the microwave and stir in the puffed rice cereal, mixing to coat.
5. Pour the puffed rice mixture over the chunky peanut butter layer in the baking dish and press flat. Refrigerate for at least 30 minutes. Remove then cut into squares.

Nutrition:

Calories: 977

Fat: 66 g

Carbs: 83 g

Protein: 26 g

Cranberry Orange Pound Cake

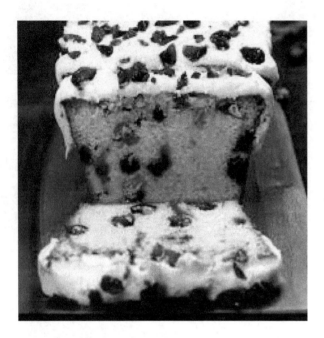

Preparation time: 15 minutes

Cooking time: 50 minutes

Servings: 6-8

Ingredients:

- 2 cups fresh cranberries
- 2 tablespoons, plus 1 1/3 cups sugar, divided
- 1 cup plain coconut yogurt
- 1 large banana, mashed
- 2 teaspoons grated orange zest
- 1 teaspoon vanilla extract
- ½ cup vegetable oil
- 1½ cups all-purpose flour
- 2 teaspoons baking powder
- ½ teaspoon salt
- 1/3 cup, plus 2 tablespoons freshly squeezed orange juice
- 1 cup powdered sugar

Directions:

1. Preheat the oven to 350°F. Grease a standard-size loaf pan. Line the bottom with parchment paper lengthwise, letting some hang over the edges. Set aside.

2. Mix the cranberries and 2 tablespoons of granulated sugar in a food processor or blender until coarsely chopped. Set aside.

3. In a large bowl, whisk together the yogurt, 1 cup of sugar, the banana, orange zest, vanilla extract, and oil. Stir in the cranberry mixture.

4. Mix the flour, baking powder, plus salt in a medium bowl. Incorporate the dry mixture into the wet mixture until smooth.

5. Pour the batter into the loaf pan and bake for 50 minutes, or until a toothpick inserted in the center comes out clean.

6. While the cake bakes, make the orange simple syrup. Mix the rest of the 1/3 cup of sugar plus 1/3 cup of orange juice in a small saucepan over medium heat. Simmer until your sugar dissolves and the syrup is clear. Set aside.

7. Remove the cake from oven and let cool for 10 minutes. Remove from the loaf pan and place on a wire rack on top of a rimmed baking sheet to catch the syrup. Pour the simple syrup over the cake. Let cool completely.

8. Make the orange glaze. Whisk the powdered sugar and the remaining 2 tablespoons of orange juice in a medium bowl until no lumps remain. Drizzle over the cooled cake. Serve and store leftovers in an airtight container.

Nutrition:

Calories: 536

Fat: 15 g

Carbs: 99 g

Protein: 3 g

Strawberry Rhubarb Coffee Cake

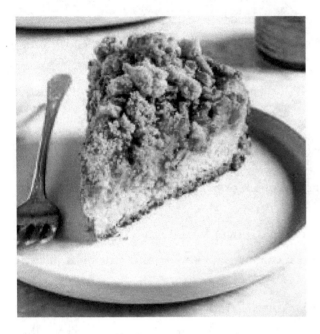

Preparation time: 15 minutes

Cooking time: 45 minutes

Servings: 6-8

Ingredients:

For the filling:

- 2 cups rhubarb, thinly sliced
- 2 cups strawberries, sliced
- 1 tablespoon lemon juice
- 2/3 cup granulated sugar
- 3 tablespoons cornstarch

For the cake:

- 1½ cups all-purpose flour
- ¼ teaspoon baking soda
- 1 teaspoon baking powder
- ¼ teaspoon salt
- ¼ cup vegan butter, softened
- ¾ cup granulated sugar

- ½ cup coconut yogurt
- 1 banana, mashed
- 1 teaspoon vanilla extract

For the topping:

- ¾ cup all-purpose flour
- ½ cup granulated sugar
- ½ teaspoon ground cinnamon
- ¼ teaspoon ground nutmeg
- 5 tablespoons melted butter

Directions:

1. For the filling, set a medium saucepan over medium heat. Add the rhubarb, strawberries, lemon juice, sugar, and cornstarch and stir to combine.
2. Simmer, then adjust to low and continue simmering until thickened, stirring often, for 5 to 7 minutes. Remove the filling from heat and let cool.
3. For the cake, preheat the oven to 350°F. Mix the flour, baking soda, baking powder, plus salt in a small bowl. Set aside.
4. Combine the butter plus sugar using an electric hand mixer and a large bowl or a stand mixer with the paddle attachment and beat on high until light and fluffy, about 5 minutes.
5. Put the yogurt, banana, plus vanilla extract and beat until combined. Adjust the speed to low then slowly add the dry mixture until fully incorporated.
6. Pour the batter evenly into a prepared 9-inch springform pan. Top with cooled strawberry-rhubarb filling and set aside.
7. For the topping, combine the flour, sugar, cinnamon, nutmeg, and butter in a medium bowl. Stir to form a crumble topping. Sprinkle evenly over the filling.
8. Bake within 45 minutes or until a toothpick inserted in the center comes out clean and the topping is browned. Let cool for 10 minutes and serve or store in an airtight container.

Nutrition:

Calories: 479

Fat: 14 g

Carbs: 86 g

Protein: 5 g

Apple Crumble

Preparation time: 15 minutes

Cooking time: 25 minutes

Servings: 6

Ingredients:

For the filling:

- 4 to 5 apples, cored and chopped (about 6 cups)
- ½ cup unsweetened applesauce, or ¼ cup water
- 2 to 3 tablespoons unrefined sugar (coconut, date, sucanat, maple syrup)
- 1 teaspoon ground cinnamon
- Pinch sea salt

For the crumble:

- 2 tablespoons almond butter, or cashew or sunflower seed butter
- 2 tablespoons maple syrup
- 1½ cups rolled oats
- ½ cup walnuts, finely chopped
- ½ teaspoon ground cinnamon
- 2 to 3 tablespoons unrefined granular sugar (coconut, date, sucanat)

Directions:

1. Preheat the oven to 350°F. Put the apples and applesauce in an 8-inch-square baking dish, and sprinkle with the sugar, cinnamon, and salt. Toss to combine.
2. In a medium bowl, mix together the nut butter and maple syrup until smooth and creamy. Add the oats, walnuts, cinnamon, and sugar and stir to coat, using your hands if necessary.
3. Sprinkle the topping over the apples, and put the dish in the oven. Bake for 20 to 25 minutes, or until the fruit is soft and the topping is lightly browned.

Nutrition:

Calories: 356

Fat: 17g

Carbs: 49g

Protein: 7g

Cashew-Chocolate Truffles

Preparation time: 15 minutes

Cooking time: 0 minutes

Servings: 12

Ingredients:

- 1 cup raw cashews, soaked/dipped in water overnight
- ¾ cup pitted dates
- 2 tablespoons coconut oil
- 1 cup unsweetened shredded coconut, divided
- 1 to 2 tablespoons cocoa powder, to taste

Directions:

1. In a food processor, combine the cashews, dates, coconut oil, ½ cup of shredded coconut, and cocoa powder.
2. Pulse until fully incorporated; it will resemble chunky cookie dough. Spread the remaining ½ cup of shredded coconut on a plate.
3. Form the mixture into tablespoon-size balls and roll on the plate to cover with the shredded coconut. Transfer to a parchment paper–lined plate or baking sheet. Repeat to make 12 truffles.
4. Place the truffles in the refrigerator for 1 hour to set. Transfer the truffles to a storage container or freezer-safe bag and seal.

Nutrition:

Calories 238

Fat: 18g

Protein: 3g

Carbohydrates: 16g

Chapter 6. 14 Days Meal Plan For Pegan Diet

Days	Breakfast	Lunch	Dinner	Dessert
1	BREAKFAST PALEO MUFFINS	TANGY BROCCOLI SALAD	SWEET POTATO BISQUE	TART APPLE GRANITA
2	PALEO BANANA PANCAKES	SUMMER ROLLS WITH PEANUT SAUCE	CHICKPEA MEDLEY	LEMON-LIME SHERBET
3	PLANTAIN PANCAKES	CHEESY WHITE BEAN CAULIFLOWER SOUP	PASTA WITH LEMON AND ARTICHOKES	PAVLOVA WITH PEACHES
4	SWEET POTATO WAFFLES	SPLIT PEA SOUP	ROASTED PINE NUT ORZO	TROPICAL VANILLA SNOW CONE
5	ORANGE AND DATES GRANOLA	QUINOA & CHICKPEA TABBOULEH	BANANA AND ALMOND BUTTER OATS	PEANUT BUTTER, NUT, AND FRUIT COOKIES
6	BREAKFAST BURRITO	CAULIFLOWER CAESAR SALAD WITH CHICKPEA CROUTONS	RED TOFU CURRY	CHOCOLATE COVERED DATES
7	SPINACH FRITTATA	VEGETABLE ROSE POTATO	SPICY TOMATO-LENTIL STEW	HOT CHOCOLATE
8	SQUASH BLOSSOM FRITTATA	RICE ARUGULA SALAD	MIXED-BEAN CHILI	VANILLA CUPCAKES

9	BREAKFAST BURGER	TOMATO SALAD	BUTTERNUT SQUASH SOUP	STUFFED DRIED FIGS
10	GREEN BREAKFAST SMOOTHIE	KALE APPLE ROASTED ROOT VEGETABLE SALAD	SPLIT-PEA SOUP	FETA CHEESECAKE
11	WARM MAPLE AND CINNAMON QUINOA	RICE ARUGULA SALAD WITH SESAME GARLIC DRESSING	TOMATO BISQUE	PEAR CROUSTADE
12	BLUEBERRY AND CHIA SMOOTHIE	ROASTED LEMON ASPARAGUS WATERCRESS SALAD	CHEESY POTATO-BROCCOLI SOUP	MELOMAKARONA
13	APPLE AND CINNAMON OATMEAL	PUMPKIN AND BRUSSELS SPROUTS MIX	VEGETABLE STEW	LOUKOUMADES (FRIED HONEY BALLS)
14	SPICED ORANGE BREAKFAST COUSCOUS	ALMOND AND TOMATO SALAD	FRIJOLES DE LA OLLA	CRÈME CARAMEL

Standard Us/Metric Measurement Conversions

VOLUME CONVERSIONS

US Volume Measure	Metric Equivalent
$1/8$ teaspoon	0.5 milliliter
$1/4$ teaspoon	1 milliliter
$1/2$ teaspoon	2 milliliters
1 teaspoon	5 milliliters
$1/2$ tablespoon	7 milliliters
1 tablespoon (3 teaspoons)	15 milliliters
2 tablespoons (1 fluid ounce)	30 milliliters
$1/4$ cup (4 tablespoons)	60 milliliters
$1/3$ cup	90 milliliters
$1/2$ cup (4 fluid ounces)	125 milliliters
$2/3$ cup	160 milliliters
$3/4$ cup (6 fluid ounces)	180 milliliters
1 cup (16 tablespoons)	250 milliliters
1 pint (2 cups)	500 milliliters
1 quart (4 cups)	1 liter (about)

WEIGHT CONVERSIONS

US Weight Measure	Metric Equivalent
$^1/_2$ ounce	15 grams
1 ounce	30 grams
2 ounces	60 grams
3 ounces	85 grams
$^1/_4$ pound (4 ounces)	115 grams
$^1/_2$ pound (8 ounces)	225 grams
$^3/_4$ pound (12 ounces)	340 grams
1 pound (16 ounces)	454 grams

OVEN TEMPERATURE CONVERSIONS

Degrees Fahrenheit	Degrees Celsius
200 degrees F	95 degrees C
250 degrees F	120 degrees C
275 degrees F	135 degrees C
300 degrees F	150 degrees C
325 degrees F	160 degrees C
350 degrees F	180 degrees C
375 degrees F	190 degrees C
400 degrees F	205 degrees C
425 degrees F	220 degrees C
450 degrees F	230 degrees C

BAKING PAN SIZES

American	Metric
8 × 1^1/$_2$ inch round baking pan	20 × 4 cm cake tin
9 × 1^1/$_2$ inch round baking pan	23 × 3.5 cm cake tin
11 × 7 × 1^1/$_2$ inch baking pan	28 × 18 × 4 cm baking tin
13 × 9 × 2 inch baking pan	30 × 20 × 5 cm baking tin
2 quart rectangular baking dish	30 × 20 × 3 cm baking tin
15 × 10 × 2 inch baking pan	30 × 25 × 2 cm baking tin (Swiss roll tin)
9 inch pie plate	22 × 4 or 23 × 4 cm pie plate
7 or 8 inch springform pan	18 or 20 cm springform or loose bottom cake tin
9 × 5 × 3 inch loaf pan	23 × 13 × 7 cm or 2 lb narrow loaf or pate tin
1^1/$_2$ quart casserole	1.5 liter casserole
2 quart casserole	2 liter casserole

Conclusion

The Pegan diet is a hybrid diet that incorporates the best of both Paleo and Vegan diets. The Pegan diet is promoted by Dr Mark Hyman, who is a family doctor and director of the Cleveland Clinic's Centre for Functional Medicine. The pegan diet is a new fad diet that combines the paleo diet with veganism. The pegan diet requires you to eliminate all meat and animal products from your diet, while at the same time eating a large number of vegetables and plants.

The vegan diet is very advantageous as it reduces the risk of developing obesity, certain cancers, and type II diabetes. However, the diet falls short of certain amino acids that are the building blocks for proteins, which can only be achieved through diet. Moreover, it is deficient in iron, calcium, zinc, and vitamin B12.

For some individuals, a strict Paleo diet is too heavy and expensive to follow. It is also problematic when you consider health issues. Veganism, on the other hand, is equally restrictive and quite a challenge for people to stick to. Hence the integration of these two highly opposing diets, the Pegan diet, a perfect mixture of healthy benefits and few limitations makes a lot of sense for those of us who want to follow a healthy lifestyle and agree to add a limited amount of animal-based proteins in their diet.   .

You should avoid processed foods like sodas and grains found in prepared foods – including bread and other baked goods. These substances simply don't benefit our bodies in any way whatsoever! You should focus on eating whole foods from all parts of the plant kingdom, including vegetables, fruits, nuts and seeds. You can consume unsaturated oils (e.g., olive oil) because these are good for our hearts rather than refined oils (e.g., fry oil). And be sure to avoid anything fried!

The time to cook the recipe can be something better. It makes you think about the meal before you start cooking and you need to be patient about cooking. In the time of making, you can take time to relax, and you can make a portion of good food for others by the time. There will be no meal wasted.

Following the instruction, you will be able to cook well, and it will make your dinner more delicious and of higher quality. Some recipes can be fun and healthy, as well. You can make your dinner more special by making a different recipe on your own. In this case, there will be no other recipes that you can make the same things as yours. You can make different flavors and different food you can ever eat.

Simple instructions give you a bit more instruction about the ingredients, and you need to be patient to make vegan food. The steps of the recipe are well described, and if you want to better food, you can follow them carefully.

The time to be patient to make a portion of good food is one of the important ways to make a good recipe. You need to follow the instruction in the recipe below. Live a healthy life by following the recipe for better health.

I hope you have learned something!

CPSIA information can be obtained
at www.ICGtesting.com
Printed in the USA
BVHW010538200421
605286BV00021B/76